D0718882

Overcome Your
Postnatal
Depression

Hodder Arnold

A MEMBER OF THE HODDER HEADLINE GROUP

Overcome Your
Postnatal
Depression

Alice Muir
Edited by Denise Robertson

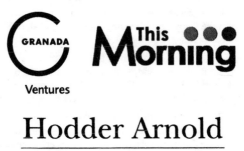

Ventures

Hodder Arnold

A MEMBER OF THE HODDER HEADLINE GROUP

Orders: Please contact Bookpoint Ltd, 130 Milton Park, Abingdon, Oxon OX14 4SB. Telephone: +44 (0) 1235 827720. Fax: +44 (0) 1235 400454. Lines are open 09.00 to 5.00, Monday to Saturday, with a 24-hour message answering service. You can also order through our website www.hoddereducation.co.uk.

British Library Cataloguing in Publication Data
A catalogue record for this title is available from the British Library.

ISBN-13: 978 0 340 94324 3

First published   2007
Impression number 10 9 8 7 6 5 4 3 2 1
Year   2012 2011 2010 2009 2008 2007

Typeset by Transet Limited, Coventry, England.
Printed in Great Britain for Hodder Education, a division of Hodder Headline, an Hachette Livre UK Company, 338 Euston Road, London, NW1 3BH, by Cox & Wyman Ltd, Reading, Berkshire.

Hodder Headline's policy is to use papers that are natural, renewable and recyclable products and made from wood grown in sustainable forests. The logging and manufacturing processes are expected to conform to the environmental regulations of the country of origin.

ABOUT THE AUTHORS

Alice Muir is a trained teacher, university lecturer and chartered psychologist. Through 25 years working with women's groups and as a trainer, counsellor and Life Coach, she has helped many women resolve emotional, health or confidence issues. As a writer she has provided expert comment to a wide variety of women's magazines and other lifestyle publications, and her books include *Make Your Sensitivity Work for You* (2006) and *Coping with a Stressed Nervous System* (2005), both published by Sheldon Press.

Denise Robertson's television career began with *BBC Breakfast Time* in 1984. She has been the resident agony aunt of ITV's *This Morning* for the last 20 years. In that time she has received over 200,000 letters covering a wide range of problems from viewers and from readers of her newspaper and magazine columns. She has written 19 novels and several works of non-fiction. Her autobiography, *Agony: Don't Get Me Started,* was published in paperback by Little Books in July 2007. She is associated with many charities, among them Relate, The Bubble Foundation, Careline and the National Council for the Divorced and Separated.

WHICH PAGE?

I think I've got postnatal depression, but how can I be sure? *Turn to page 14*

I'm having trouble explaining how I feel to my partner. *Turn to page 52*

I live on my own and everything is getting on top of me. *Turn to page 55*

I'm worried I'm not bonding with my baby. *Turn to pages 72 and 174*

I feel so angry all the time when I know I should be feeling happy. *Turn to pages 68 and 155*

I don't like the idea of taking medication because I'm breastfeeding my baby. *Turn to page 132*

I've completely gone off sex and my partner is finding this difficult. *Turn to page 195*

I'm worried about having another baby in case I get depressed again. *Turn to page 207*

To my daughter Cathy and my son Colin,
who give me endless joy and
immeasurable fulfilment.

CONTENTS

FOREWORD

By Fern Britton and Phillip Schofield

As presenters of ITV's *This Morning*, over many years we have met many incredible people with many incredible stories to tell. What we have learnt is that life can be wonderful but it can also be very hard.

Our phone-ins have generated thousands of calls a day from viewers all over Great Britain looking for suitable advice on a range of subjects. What is very obvious from these calls is that we are not alone with the personal challenges we often face and there is a great need for help in dealing with them. We are always cheered by the follow-up letters and emails from viewers saying how our experts' advice has helped them to turn their lives around.

Over the 20 years *This Morning* has been on air, Denise Robertson, our agony aunt, has regularly offered support and advice to millions of viewers on a huge range of personal problems and she spends even more time off-screen answering letters, calling those in distress and dealing with questions via the internet. As a result she is uniquely qualified to edit these books which reflect the common sense and sensitive advice that we provide on the show.

We believe these survival guides will help you to deal with the practical and emotional fallout caused by issues such as bereavement, relationship break-ups, debt, infertility, addiction, domestic violence and depression.

If you feel that your particular problems are insurmountable – don't! There is always a way to improve your life or at least get yourself on a path towards a new start. If you think you are alone with your problem – don't! Our experience shows that many of us face the same problems but are often reluctant to admit it. You have already made a great start by picking up this book.

We both wish you all the strength and support you need to tackle your own personal problems and sincerely hope we can help through these books and through our continued work on the programme.

INTRODUCTION

The worst things about postnatal depression (PND) are that you don't expect it and you don't deserve it. Added to this, the other people in your life don't expect it either and, unless they're saints, won't like its intrusion into their lives. They'll say things like 'How can you be miserable with that lovely baby lying there? Look at the little darling, it's as good as gold'. They'll ignore the fact that the little darling probably kept you awake all night and refuses to feed, and mutter darkly about 'bonding' and shake their heads in disapproval. Even worse, they'll shame you with a sad story about someone else's failed pregnancy and that can be the last straw when you already feel that life is a deep black hole from which there is no escape.

As for partners, that sane, capable rock who shared your life pre-pregnancy may now view the longed-for baby as a deadly virus which has ruined his life and turned his lover into a snivelling wreck. And just when you've accepted that your tummy muscles are now worn-out knicker elastic, you can't remember your middle name and you've let a pan boil dry because you can't do one thing at once let alone three, you open a magazine and see a glowing, celebrity mother and baby, proving that you are the **only** woman in the world who is a **failure**.

Okay. That's the downside to PND. Can there possibly be an upside? The answer is a resounding 'Yes'. PND is a recognized condition which responds well to treatment. The qualified people caring for you will have met it many times before and know exactly what to do for you. And, once they understand what's going on, no intelligent person will think it's your fault – and that includes you. Your partner, once he grasps that civilized life as we know it can be restored eventually, will return to being your rock and will be a dab hand with the nappies to boot. Before long you'll see that black hole turning first to charcoal and then to grey and eventually vanishing altogether.

The other good news is that this book has been assembled to give you all the information and support you need to make that journey back to a life worth living. It's written with both the couple and the single mum in mind. It will explode the myths about bonding and much else, and explain many of the things you, and your family, now find incomprehensible. It will also let you see that other women, famous and unknown, have experienced exactly the same thing and gone on to be happy once more. Read on and be assured that once your PND is dealt with, one of life's most wonderful experiences lies ahead.

Denise Robertson

Part 1:
What to Do
Right Now

1

There is light at the end of the tunnel

Right now, you may be feeling tired and guilty, and maybe a little puzzled and disappointed at what's been happening to you. Everything has turned out so differently from what you were expecting. You may be wondering if you'll ever feel well and happy again. We can assure you right from the start that you can get better and be your old cheerful self again. And, just as importantly, you can regain a happy and loving relationship with your baby and your partner. We will also show you that none of this is your fault, and you don't need to feel so responsible and ashamed. You're doing absolutely the right thing in reading this book. You will never regret it.

Your survival tips

- You are not alone.

- Many, many other mothers are feeling just like you, right now.

- We understand how you are feeling.

- You can and will get better.

What we are going to do in the first part of the book is begin to give you back a feeling of control over your life – something which you may feel you have lost completely. We will also get you started on the road to recovery and help you to gain a better understanding of how you have been feeling. Other women will share their own experiences with you too, and you'll find that many of them have felt very much as you are feeling now. So be assured that **you are not alone**. Be assured, too, that there is so much that you can do to make things better. We will give you lots of information about this too. However, before all that, here are some 'survival tips' for you to read right now. You may like to look back over these whenever you feel you need some reassurance.

What are the 'baby blues'?

You will probably have heard of the 'baby blues', and may know someone who has experienced this. Many women find that on the third, fourth or fifth day after their baby is born, they feel a sudden change in their mood, and begin to feel a bit weepy, irritable and down. One day you are brimming with pride and confidence, but the next your confidence suddenly disappears and everything seems like another mountain to climb. All can have been going wonderfully well, when suddenly you just can't see the point of it all any more. The joy of it escapes you completely. Tears seem to tumble out for the very slightest of reasons. Perhaps the baby's bottle is too warm or too cold, or you can't get the baby to fix on to your nipple if you're breastfeeding. Your neighbour pops in to see you, and you see her eyes taking in the untidy mess that used to be your neatly organized home. Or, more confusing, tears can well up for no reason at all. You find yourself sitting moping and can only think of negative things about having a baby.

This is the 'baby blues' and it is extremely common. Staff at the hospital, as well as your midwife, doctor and health visitor, will know all about it, and will be on the look out for it happening to you, so don't be scared to tell them how you're feeling or ask them about it. No one's really sure, but baby blues may be brought on by the hormone changes during and immediately following the birth, especially at the time when your milk comes in for the baby. You don't need any treatment for it, and it will usually disappear just as mysteriously as it arrived. What you will need is patience and understanding from those around you.

> *MYTH: Postnatal depression always comes on within a few weeks of having your baby.*
>
> **FACT:** Postnatal depression can appear at any time up to around six months after the birth.

How do you know if it's the baby blues?

Over half of new mothers will experience the 'baby blues', so you will not be alone. With it being so common, it's almost considered as normal. The most obvious way to tell if you have the baby blues is by how long the feelings last after the baby is born. If you feel completely yourself again after a few days, it will have been the baby blues. If you are still feeling down after the tenth day or so, you may be experiencing another very common condition, called postnatal depression, or PND for short.

MYTH: Postnatal depression is just the 'baby blues'.

FACT: Postnatal depression isn't 'just' anything. It's a very distressing illness affecting lots of new mothers every day. It is not the same as the baby blues, which is also an unpleasant way to feel.

What is postnatal depression?

Postnatal depression (PND) is a depression which can affect you after the birth of your baby but, unlike the baby blues which are short-lived, it continues after the first week or so. It is quite different from the baby blues and affects about one in ten of new mothers. You will probably have heard about depression or you may even have had depression yourself, or have a friend or a relative who has. Having said that, you may not actually be feeling depressed. So you may have been wondering if you really do have PND. How can you have PND if you don't feel depressed?

The thing is that feeling really low or down is just one of many ways that PND can show itself. There are all sorts of ways that PND can affect a new mother. Most are distressing and puzzling and can be quite frightening when you've never felt that way before.

Here are some of the signs of PND. Read through them and tick any of them that you can identify with:

❑ Being unusually irritable.

❑ Feeling tired and with no motivation to do anything.

❑ Not being able to get to sleep, even when the baby lets you.

❑ Feeling unable to cope.

❑ Feeling very low, or despondent.

❑ Having no interest in sex.

❑ Feeling cut off from things, or numb, or unable to enjoy anything.

❑ Feeling guilty about not coping, or about not loving the baby enough.

❑ Not feeling like eating, or comfort eating more than usual.

❑ Being hostile or indifferent to your baby.

- ❏ Being hostile or indifferent to your husband or partner.

- ❏ Having obsessive fears and worries about yourself, the baby, or members of the family.

- ❏ Having panic attacks or unusual anxiety.

- ❏ Having poor concentration.

- ❏ Finding you have problems with the simplest of decisions.

- ❏ Thinking that nothing is any good, and that there is no hope.

- ❏ Having thoughts about death.

- ❏ Waking early in the morning, before the baby wakes you.

- ❏ Wanting to cry all the time, or especially in the mornings or evenings.

- ❏ Worrying about harming yourself.

- ❏ Worrying about harming the baby.

Q. Will I ever feel better again?

A. It will take a bit of time, maybe a few weeks or months perhaps, but you will feel gradually better, yes. Just understanding what is happening to you will probably make you feel a bit better straight away.

How did you get on? Some mums with PND will pick out just one or two, others will tick almost all of them. There's no set pattern and you may have only slight problems with some, but real difficulties with another. You may have only slight trouble in making decisions, but find that you cannot concentrate at all any more, or that your relationship with your partner is at serious risk because you can't control your anger towards him.

Don't jump to conclusions just yet. Sometimes new mums can simply lack confidence in themselves as mothers. If you've never handled a baby before, let alone had to cope with everything else that goes with having one, you may be feeling quite naturally anxious and frustrated because you don't feel on top of things any more. There is a lot to looking after a baby, and you have to learn very quickly, while trying to keep the everyday routine at home going. This may be your first baby, and it's all very new and strange. You may have step-children in the house whose lives still need to go on. You may be experiencing stress and exhaustion because of these and other factors.

In addition, problems such as tiredness, disturbed sleep, poor appetite and a reduced sex drive are common and normal for a while after childbirth and, on their own, may not mean that you are depressed.

How do you know for sure if you have PND?

If it is more than two weeks since your baby was born and you've ticked one or more of the signs in the list (see pages 11–12), and these have lasted more than a few days, you should make an appointment to see your doctor. You may not have PND, but it is worth checking out exactly what's going on. Even if you haven't ticked anything on the list, but you just have a feeling that you're not yourself, or something's not quite right, then make an appointment anyway. The doctor will not mind you going along to see him, even if he finds out that you are absolutely fine and that nothing is amiss. He will be quite happy to have a satisfied customer. He'd much rather you did that than not go, and then develop something more serious later on because it wasn't dealt with at the start. Doctors are there to help you. That said, if you still feel that you'd rather speak to someone separate from your life and family, you'll find a list of helplines in Part 5, Chapter 16.

The only way to be sure if you have PND is to talk to your doctor, your health visitor, or your midwife. Try to go without the baby, so that you have a chance to talk. Take your partner or a female friend or relative with you if you need a bit of support. If you are finding it hard to leave the house or can't get a childminder, you can phone and ask your health visitor to visit you at home. She will come and have a talk with you, and may ask you to complete a simple questionnaire like the one you've just done. If you don't feel up to filling out the questionnaire, you will be asked the questions and the doctor or health visitor will complete it for you. They will then tell you if they think you have PND and explain how they can help you. We'll tell you much more about how the doctor and health visitor can help you in Part 2 of the book, but you should make an appointment now if you identify with any of these signs, or if you are worried in any way.

Worries about harming yourself or the baby

If you are having any thoughts about harming yourself or the baby, don't panic, and don't think you are going mad. These thoughts are extremely common and hardly ever lead to you actually carrying them out. They are a very unpleasant part of having PND but we assure you, having a thought, any thought, does not mean that you will carry out that thought.

If you are having any worrying thoughts like this, make an appointment to see your doctor straight away, today. The sooner you have some help with your feelings, the sooner they will disappear. If you do feel there is any chance at all that you may carry out these thoughts, you must tell someone straight away, now. Call the doctor and tell the person who answers the call. They will understand and they will be able to help you.

MYTH: If you think you will harm your baby, you probably will.

FACT: It is extremely rare for a new mum to harm her baby. It is extremely common to have thoughts like these, but having them doesn't mean that you'll carry them out.

How are you feeling right now

As you read this, you are most likely to be feeling worried and exhausted, with any number of the signs of PND from the list on pages 11–12. Added to this it's all been such a surprise to you. You had been so looking forward to the baby coming, and yet now it all seems more like a nightmare than the wonderful dreams you had before the birth. You may have had a difficult pregnancy or a difficult birth, too, and still be tired and sore, and not physically your usual self. You may have a wound still healing from the birth or from a caesarian section, with all the complications and concerns that this can bring. If you are breastfeeding, you will be worrying about how this will all affect your milk supply. Will you have enough for the next feed? Sometimes you have more than enough, and sometimes it's a struggle, and your baby has to work so hard to satisfy her hunger. Your baby may be poorly, or still in hospital after the birth, which will naturally make you even more anxious. Tick any of the items in the list on page 18 which apply to you right now.

- ❏ Are you feeling guilty and ashamed?

- ❏ Do you worry about how this is affecting the baby and your other children?

- ❏ Are you scared people will think you are a bad mother?

- ❏ Are you scared you'll do something terrible?

- ❏ Are you terrified that you're going mad?

- ❏ Are you scared they'll take away your baby?

- ❏ Do you feel that you want this nightmare to go away; to be living the wonderful dreams you had before the birth?

- ❏ Are you angry with what life has thrown at you?

- ❏ Do you want to be coping like everybody else?

- ❏ Do you want the old 'you' back?

You may also be feeling guilty about how you are affecting the lives of everybody around you. You just want life to get back to normal again. But how? This is all new territory for you and you've no idea what to do for the best. You used to be such an organized person, holding down a responsible job, and now the simplest of decisions or difficulties is totally beyond you, and you sometimes just want to go back to bed and hide under the covers till it all goes away. What has happened to the old you?

Be reassured: things can and will get better

We can assure you that you are not going mad and that most people with depression do get better. There is also so much that you can do to help yourself and those around you. We know you are so tired and so discouraged, and it can all seem like such a huge effort. Even reading this book is a strain. However, if you stick with it, we promise that we will help you to find that energy from deep inside yourself and we will show you in a straightforward way what exactly you can do to make things better. Starting from today. Starting right now.

Q. I've been feeling like this for months now. Does that mean it will take me longer to get better?

A. It shouldn't make any difference. The time taken to recover fully does vary, but it shouldn't matter how long you've had PND to begin with.

Stop worrying

You can begin by trying not to worry so much about everything. And we know that is easy to say, but not so easy to do, but we'll give you lots of help with this. PND can make you feel anxious and worried about everything and anything.

There may be particular worries going through your mind just now, such as being scared that your baby might be taken into care if you can't get things together. Being afraid like this sometimes stops a mother asking for the help she needs, especially if she is on her own. Be reassured, it is only very, very occasionally that a baby is taken into care, and this is seen very much as a last resort. The authorities see supporting the mother and the family as the best way they can help, not by taking the baby away.

You may also be worried about bonding with your baby. You may be concerned that how you are feeling and behaving might be affecting this. We will give you plenty of help with this, too, later in this book. Armed with this know-how, you will be able to make that bond as strong as it can be. For now, even if it's difficult for you, spend lots of time in close physical contact with your baby, making eye contact and talking. Even if you don't feel like it, going through the motions will help build the bond.

Another worry you might have is how this is affecting your partner and any other children you may have. Having any kind of illness will impact on your close family but an illness like PND, which many people don't really understand, can impact all the more. We will help you with this so relax, we are here now working with you on this. **You don't have to carry all of that heavy burden by yourself any more.** We will share it with you, until you can manage on your own.

Three important things to remember

The first thing to remember is that **none of this is your fault**. It is not happening because you are weak or stupid or going mad, and it's not happening because of something you could have done, or should have done better. It's not because you didn't go to the antenatal classes as often as you meant to. It's not because you didn't do all those exercises and read all those books, which were recommended to you. Nor is it because of something you did or maybe shouldn't have done, such as those occasional glasses of wine, or that special cream you were meant to rub on your bump every day, or the music to play to the baby in the womb. No, none of this is down to any of these things, or to you. PND is thought to be caused mainly by the total upheaval in your life, which pregnancy, and the birth and arrival of a new baby brings about. This isn't something which you have any control over, so stop blaming yourself and concentrate on getting yourself well again. We'll tell you how in this book.

The next important thing to remember is that **you are not alone**. You may feel completely alone – even in a room full of people you can feel totally isolated, with no one seeming to

Q. Can't I sort this out for myself? Do I need to see a doctor?

A. If you suspect you have PND, you should definitely talk to your doctor, midwife or health visitor. PND will get better eventually on its own, but this will take a long time, and there's no need for you and your family to suffer like that for so long.

understand or care – but people around you really do want to help. They are just not sure how, and they don't know what to say or do. There are also many, many other women who have felt the way you do now, or felt that way in the past. They understand more than most and we'll tell you in Chapter 9 how you can tap into that army of support if you want to. And of course, there's us, and this book. We are totally on your side and walking along beside you.

The third thing to remember is that **there is so much you can do to help yourself**. We will take you through all of these things and we'll do it in manageable chunks, as we know that you may be finding it so hard to concentrate on anything right now. Even finding the time to read this book will be difficult. Do try to make the time, even if it's just five minutes here and five minutes there. You won't regret it. Don't hesitate to use a pen or 'stickies' to highlight or underline the bits you find most useful, so that you can easily find them when you need them. It can be so hard to remember even the simplest of things.

Three tips to help you right now

It will take you time to speak to your doctor or health visitor, but what can you do now, right this minute? Here are some things you can do straight away to help you to feel a little better:

- Slowly take a long and deep breath in, then let it out with a sigh, letting any tension in your body gradually go with it. Now do that again, slowly, no rush.

- If your appetite is poor, make sure you eat something little and often, even if you don't feel like it. It doesn't matter what you eat at this stage – anything will help – low blood sugar through not eating can make you feel anxious, tired, shaky, moody and panicky.

- Stop worrying about what the house looks like. It really doesn't matter for now. As long as it is functional, all the rest can wait. Don't try to be superwoman – concentrate on you and the baby and the rest will slip into place later on.

I thought I was losing my mind. I was sure of it. Then I heard a discussion on the radio and realized they were talking about exactly how I felt. Such a weight off my mind. It wasn't just me after all. I went to see my doctor later that week and I've never looked back.

Julie, 28

It was such a shock when I had my little girl three months ago. I had the 'baby blues' and everybody told me that it would pass within a day or two. But it didn't, it just got worse and worse. I've never felt anything like it before. I was so relieved when my health visitor told me I wasn't going mad and she could help me.

Rona, 36

2

How those around you are feeling right now

In Chapter 1, we concentrated quite rightly on you and how you are feeling. We hope we have given you clear explanations and options on where to go from here. However, as you will know only too well, postnatal depression (PND) doesn't just affect the person who has it – it also impacts strongly on everybody around you, from your baby, to your nearest loved ones, to your neighbours and friends. They will all have noticed a change in you too. In this chapter we will try to give you some insight into how they might be feeling, and this may allow you to see their behaviour and reactions in a new light. In Chapter 4, there is a section for them to read if you want them to, but more on that later. First, some more 'survival tips' just for you.

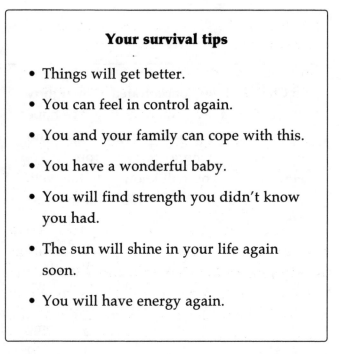

Your survival tips

- Things will get better.

- You can feel in control again.

- You and your family can cope with this.

- You have a wonderful baby.

- You will find strength you didn't know you had.

- The sun will shine in your life again soon.

- You will have energy again.

Your partner

If you are living with a partner, he will probably be feeling guilty and finding it really hard to cope, too. He may not know what to say and he won't know what to do to help you. He may feel that his once friendly and loving wife or girlfriend has just disappeared and he has a new irritable version in her place. So you may be having more frequent and more heated arguments

MYTH: If you don't bond with your baby in the first 24–48 hours, you never will bond properly.

FACT: Love sometimes takes time to grow and you can still 'fall in love' with your baby weeks after the birth.

than usual. Or, you may be communicating less and less, as he just doesn't know what to say and is scared he upsets you by getting it wrong. You may feel that he just doesn't understand.

It may help you to know that **men often want to fix a problem and do practical things to help you, rather than talk about it**. So don't be too upset if he seems to be offering to put up shelves, fix the washing machine or do the dishes, rather than just sit down, give you a much needed cuddle and talk it over with you. It's just his way of dealing with the problem as he sees it.

He may even start searching the internet for information about postnatal illness and not want to tell you in case he upsets you. So don't be too surprised if he suddenly closes the window on the screen or turns the computer off when you come into the room. He may even phone NHS (National Health Service) Direct for help when you are out or start reading your women's magazines when he thinks you're not looking.

> *MYTH: People with depression are just weak people who can't cope with life.*
>
> **FACT:** This is absolute nonsense. Depression and PND can happen to anyone, whatever their strengths and weaknesses. Sir Winston Churchill, who was such a brave and capable prime minister during the Second World War, had frequent bouts of depression.

Many men find talking about feelings really difficult to do. It's just that they are wired differently from us women. We'll give you some help in coping with that in Chapter 4. On the other hand, some men are really quite good at this sort of thing and may even be raising the subject with you that something is wrong and suggesting you may have PND. You may be resistant to this idea or maybe that's why you are reading this book now.

Sometimes men cope by simply ignoring the problem, denying there is anything to worry about at all and avoiding talking about it. Your partner may be going out more than usual and coming back late as well as switching off his mobile while he's out. All this can be a way of coping too. Inside he will be just as scared, confused and upset as you are. Still waters really can run extremely deep.

Your partner may be reacting in many different ways. He may feel any of the following:

- Worried about you.

- Guilty.

- Afraid someone will take the baby away.

- Scared and ashamed that there is a problem.

- Worried he can't cope with the responsibility of it all.

- Exhausted caring for you and your other children.

- Frustrated and helpless.

- Disappointed or angry at what has happened.

- Resentful that everything was great before the baby came and spoiled things.

- Blame towards the baby.

- Resentful that his needs are being ignored.

- Resentful of the time you spend with the baby.

- Scared you might harm yourself or the baby.

- Worried about the effect on the baby.

Your partner can feel down too

We've just been thinking about the feelings your partner may be having just now, and much of this can make him feel a bit down as well. Also, some of the reasons for you feeling down can affect your partner, and lower his mood. On top of that, he may be particularly missing having you all to himself, and the freedom you used to enjoy as a couple – being able to make love or go out anywhere, any time. Now you're too tired or too sore for sex, or you're scared it will wake the baby. If you're breastfeeding, he can't fondle your breasts the way he used to. Also, before you even take a step out of the door, there's the nappy change, feed-time, the pram, baby's jacket, blankets, bottle, changing mat, and all the rest to think about. This soon becomes second nature, but requires a bit of adjusting to and, inevitably, an experience of loss for you both. Any kind of loss can make you feel low, so to some extent, your partner is in the same boat as you, just at the other end of it.

Your other children

If you already have one or more child in the house you will be worrying about their needs as well as those of your new baby. On a positive note, they can keep you busy with their packed lunches to prepare, and the school or playgroup run to do, and this can help you keep some sense of normality in your days. However, they will be feeling worried and frightened, too. Children are like little barometers, reflecting the mood in the house. They may not say anything about this, as they won't want to upset you but it may show in their behaviour. You may find that their schoolwork deteriorates, or a usually quiet child becomes a noisy one, or a normally outgoing and chatty child becomes quiet and thoughtful. Like your partner, you may find that they've been searching the internet, trying to work out what's wrong. Children are very aware about things like PND these days, through their general reading and TV programmes.

Other mums

As soon as you are pregnant, you will come into contact with other women who are pregnant or have recently had babies. First at the doctor's clinic, then at antenatal classes and, of course, at the hospital if you've had a hospital birth. Before the birth other pregnant women will share your excitement, your aches and pains and your worries. You'll swap stories about your stretch marks, breastfeeding and nappies. When the babies are born, you may still remain friends with these new acquaintances and you may have made some friends for life. Some of your old friends will also be having babies at the same time as you are. So you will most likely have a new circle of other mums around you, which can be a support for almost anything.

It can be a bit different from stretch marks and nappies when it comes to feeling down, or any of the many other ways PND can show itself. You may not want to tell them how you are feeling, especially when you see how well they are coping and how cheerful and delighted they are. If you are brave enough to confide in one of these mums, they may well respond by saying 'How can you be feeling depressed? You have such a beautiful baby and you had such an easy birth.' So you clam up and don't say another word and you feel even worse and more guilty. After all, isn't she right? Shouldn't you be feeling over the moon? Aren't you just an ungrateful and unworthy mother not to be happy? This, in turn, will make you feel like a bad mother all the more. **Do remember, none of this is true, and none of this is your fault.** Absolutely none of it. Do also bear in mind that one of these mums may be hiding their PND, feeling ashamed and guilty, just like you are.

Q. What is a health visitor?

A. A health visitor is a very experienced nurse who has taken extra training in the care of families, including mothers and children. After you come home with your baby, and the midwife has finished her visits with you, you will have regular home visits from a health visitor. They also organize and run baby clinics at your doctor's practice.

Your mother

If you have your mother or your partner's mother nearby, this can be a huge help. Like everyone else, she may be confused and not really understand how you are feeling and may say all the wrong things. So make allowances. On the other hand, your mother may understand completely how you are feeling. Many women are very tuned in to problems like this and if she is, this will be a huge benefit to you.

If your mother has no idea what PND is like, she may say things which really upset you such as 'Why on earth are you feeling down? – you have a beautiful perfect baby.' 'Look at all those poor women who can't conceive, or those who lost their babies. How can you be feeling low compared to them?' All this really hurts and makes you feel even more wretched, more guilty and ashamed. Don't let it make you feel worse. Like we've said already, people just don't understand and they think what they are saying might help you. We know it won't, but they don't. They are trying to help, so don't be too angry with them. More on this in Chapter 4.

Remember, too, that what you are feeling may bring back unpleasant memories for your mother – she may have had PND herself. This would have been quite some time ago, when PND was not understood and recognized the way it is now. So she may never have told anyone about how she was feeling and she may well not have had any help at all with her PND. She may have been criticized and called a bad mother, or told she had to 'pull herself together for the sake of the baby'. So what you are feeling may bring back very unpleasant memories for her and she may react to you in any number of ways. She may be a super ally, understanding things better than anyone else possibly could. However, she may find the whole thing is just too painful and sensitive an area, and find being reminded of it quite traumatic. We know that this is a difficult time for you, but you may need to tread carefully with your mother and your partner's mother.

Q. I had my baby and came home all on the same day. One of the nurses told me mums used to spend a whole week in hospital. Is this true?

A. Yes, 20 to 30 years ago new mothers would spend a week in hospital following the birth of their baby, recovering, and having help learning to feed and care for the baby.

Your relationship with your mother before the baby was born will tell you a lot about how she will react to the way you are feeling now. If she has always been a close mum, and you could talk about anything, that will be such a benefit to you. If talking about feelings or moods has always been a bit of a no-go area, it may well still be, so you may find communicating with her is a problem. More on this in Chapter 4. Also, your relationship with your mother may change with the birth of a first baby. She is now a grandmother and you are a mother. You both have these changes to adapt to, and there will be corresponding adjustments to the relationship between the two of you. This can be a bit awkward and take time.

Your father

It may be that you have your father nearby, and father–daughter relationships can often be really strong. If this is the case for you, this can also be a wonderful source of support. Don't feel you can't talk to him now just because it's 'women's problems'. Just as with mums and partners, dads can react in many different ways to you having PND.

Other family and friends

Members of your family and your friends can feel quite at a loss. Even friends who've known you for a long time and close family can suddenly be quite stuck for words. If you had broken your leg or you had flu, they would know exactly how to react and what to say and do to help you. They will probably have been incredibly supportive in the past. But this is different. You are not yourself. You are acting strangely, avoiding going out perhaps or just sitting there, looking unhappy and saying very little when they come to visit.

They just don't know what to do, or what to say to help. So, sometimes, they'll say things that upset you, such as, 'How can you feel down when you have such a lovely baby?' or, 'It will all seem better in the morning' or even, 'Pull yourself together'. Family may gradually visit less, or not at all. Friends may avoid you and even dodge down another aisle in the supermarket when they see you coming. They don't mean to hurt you. They just don't understand, and they don't know how to help you.

Things people will say to try to help

Saying the wrong things

Most people, when they are faced with someone who is depressed, don't know what to say. Worse than that, they are very likely to say all the wrong things – things which will not make you feel better at all. Most people think they should try to cheer you up, so they will look for the positive things they can remind you of, and say things like, 'You're so lucky to have a partner like Simon. He's such a help.' It's not that Simon isn't a help, and it's not that you aren't aware of that, it's just that this doesn't help someone who is depressed, even if your friends think it will. It's just not as simple as that. Alternatively, they may say, 'You have such a lovely house, and all these beautiful presents for the baby.' Well-meaning neighbours may say, 'At least you have a perfect, healthy baby. Think of how you'd feel if he was disabled or had a serious medical problem, like Angela down the road.' None of these things help at all. They are more likely to make you feel much worse, even more ungrateful and even more confused and depressed.

Always remember that people don't mean to hurt you. They just don't understand and they don't know how to help you. Before you had PND, what would you have said to a friend who was feeling the way you are? It's really hard to know what it's like if you haven't experienced it. A bit like having sex, or being pregnant, really difficult to imagine if you haven't been there yourself. Reading this book will help them to understand PND better, as well as you. So, pass it on for them to read next, after you've finished it. And there's a special section in Chapter 4, just for them to read.

Q. What is a panic attack?

A. A sudden attack of severe anxiety. Panic attacks can occur up to several times a day. The symptoms can include pounding heart, sweating, trembling, shortness of breath, light-headedness and fears of dying or of 'going crazy'. They are a normal reaction of the body and are very unlikely to do you any harm, even though they feel awful.

Saying the right things

Many people will say the wrong thing, but you will find that some of those around you will say the right things, if you let them. In fact, they may not say very much at all. They may let you do the talking and just listen supportively to what you have to say. That can be such a relief. They may just sit quietly with you, just being there, if you don't feel like talking. Some people do this quite naturally – nobody has to tell them how – they just know. Others may have had a bit of training in how to be supportive and a good listener. Then there will be other mums, maybe a friend or a relative, or a neighbour, someone who has been where you are now, and knows what you are feeling. So they know what to say, and what not to say. You will find other women like these can be an incredible support. Hopefully they will make themselves known to you and will be there for you.

I had no problems when my first little boy, Jamie, was born. Felt great. Got my figure back quickly too. When my second little boy, Connor was born, it couldn't have been more difficult. I've never felt like that in my life before. It's almost impossible to explain. Hard to find the words. I thought my boyfriend, Ray, didn't understand, or didn't care. He was so quiet and just wouldn't talk to me about it at all. He just left the room if I mentioned the subject. Then one day, he just burst into tears out of the blue when we were on our way to the shops. I'd never seen him cry before. We both ended up crying together, holding each other. I didn't realize until then how it was all affecting him and how he was really feeling. Things were so much easier after that.

Becky, 29

3

More immediate help for you

In Chapter 2 we spent some time thinking about how everybody around you might be feeling and reacting to the changes in your behaviour since the baby was born. Now it's time to concentrate on you again, and this chapter will help you with the immediate situation of realizing that you might have postnatal depression (PND), or of having had it recently confirmed by the doctor. We'll help you with telling your partner and we'll show you some ways of relaxing and coping with panic attacks if you have them. We'll also give you some initial tips on how to lift your mood or cope when you are angry, as well as offering some advice about bonding with your baby. There will be much more on all of this in Part 2, but it's time to make a start on these things now. First though, some more 'survival tips' for you. Remember you can look back over these at any time.

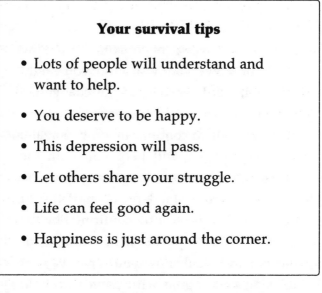

Your survival tips

- Lots of people will understand and want to help.

- You deserve to be happy.

- This depression will pass.

- Let others share your struggle.

- Life can feel good again.

- Happiness is just around the corner.

How can you tell your partner?

You may have been trying to cope with all this on your own and have bottled it all up inside. It can be easier to do this sometimes. You have been very strong and self-reliant doing this, but it's time to let things out now. This will be much better for you. Perhaps you find you are talking all the time about how you are feeling, and those around you are beginning to switch off whenever you start to talk. Whatever way you have been coping with things until now, it's time to explain things clearly to those around you.

The first person who needs to know about how you are really feeling is your partner. If you don't have a partner, you need to share this burden with your mum, dad, a sister, or your best friend. They will probably know already that something is amiss, and being able to understand things better will be a great relief to them and a great support for you.

Take time to explain things properly. Your partner will need time to absorb what you are saying, so don't rush. Find some quiet, private time, preferably when the baby is asleep. You could even get a babysitter for an hour or so to let you talk in peace. Have someone with you if you feel you need moral support and maybe have a leaflet or something from the internet ready for him to read if you think that might help him, or make things easier for you.

Remember he may need some time to take things in, so don't expect too much at first. Be ready for him to be surprised or scared or angry or whatever – there's no way of knowing how someone will react. He may just shrug his shoulders because he doesn't know what to say. So give him time to absorb the first impact and don't expect too much. Then be ready for him to keep asking you questions, or go very quiet, or maybe have mood changes for the next few days or more. We all react in different ways.

You may find that he blames himself for what is happening to you. He made you pregnant after all. Maybe he suggested a baby or maybe he wanted a baby more than you did. There are all sorts of ways in which your partner might blame himself or feel guilty. Maybe he hasn't even noticed the trouble you've been having or maybe you've been very good at hiding it. Many mums are very good at this.

If you simply feel that talking about this to your partner is beyond you, then your health visitor or doctor may be able to help you. They will explain things to your partner for you, provided you give them your permission to do this.

If you live on your own

It is difficult enough being depressed after your baby is born, but all the more difficult if you have to cope with it by yourself. Even though you have the baby with you most of the time, it will be a long time before the baby feels like company. You may be recovering from the hurt of a recently broken relationship too, or feeling guilty about having had a one-night stand and not using contraception. Maybe the baby's father is in another relationship as well as being with you. Then there is all the soul-searching you may be going through about whether or not to tell him about his new child.

You can be faced with an angry family too, either yours or his, with all the anxiety and distress that can cause. Even going out for a walk with the baby or going to get some shopping can be a nightmare, worrying about who you might bump into and the reaction you may get from them. Your life may be even more complicated and you may not be sure who the father is. Maybe he's married and you are having to share him with his wife, who knows nothing about you or the baby. All of this will just make you feel all the worse and all the more isolated and alone.

Having a new baby and living on your own is demanding enough, but it is so very hard and unfair if you also have PND to contend with. Most of the symptoms of PND are made worse by being alone for long periods of time. You are also likely to be more tired, with little time for rest and relaxation, and nobody to help out or take a turn with the night feeds. All this can just make you feel more down.

So you musn't try to go it completely alone. You don't need to soldier on and you don't need to show everybody that you can cope. PND is an illness like any other. If you were physically unwell, you wouldn't feel bad about having some help. This is no different. Your health and the baby's health matter most. We hope that, even though you live alone, there is someone around you who can, and will, be there for you. Family, friends, a neighbour, a live-out boyfriend perhaps. Make sure to invite them round if you haven't already. People love to feel wanted and they love to feel they have been able to help. Almost everybody loves a new baby to make a fuss of, so make the most of offers of help to have some precious time to yourself. If there isn't anyone there for you, you must contact a support group straight away. **You don't have to do this on your own.** There are many really excellent groups out there and they won't judge you. They will just be there for you. You'll find full contact details for these in Part 5. Go on, do it now.

More help for you

Here are four easy things you can do right now to help you to cope a little better:

- Take naps whenever you can. A five- or ten-minute catnap can be really reviving.

- Let yourself get close to your partner if you can – at least kiss and cuddle. This will comfort you both and help bring about the return of full sexual feelings sooner. Do not feel guilty if this takes some time.

- Think a positive thought whenever you can. This sounds silly, but it can really help. 'What a lovely day', 'How blue the sky is', 'It's good to be inside on a cold day like this', 'I'm glad we chose that rug', 'I feel really comfy in these slippers mum gave me'. No need to look for big positive things, a little positive thought made often each day can be very powerful in lifting your mood.

- Keep busy. You will be busy with the baby, but when you do have time on your hands, don't give in to temptation and sit down to brood in that comfy armchair or sofa. Always have to hand something to do, which doesn't need too much concentration. Anything which will take up your mind for a little while will do, be it a TV programme, a magazine to read, calls to friends, sudoku, a jigsaw or crossword puzzle, whatever you find will take up your thoughts for a while.

MYTH: People with depression are just fed up or bored.

FACT: Depression at any time of your life is a real illness. It's not the same as feeling fed up or bored. It is much deeper and long-lasting, and usually includes a profound sense of hopelessness.

Quick fix relaxation ideas

The physical tension brought about by PND can be very persistent and difficult to relieve. For many people the straightforward answer to this is to spend time doing something which helps to relax your muscles. A walk on the beach, a lazy bath, listening to music, yoga, gardening, or a physical activity such as swimming or jogging can all be relaxing depending on your own individual taste. The main thing is to take time out to do something you enjoy and which is relaxing for you.

These simple pastimes are the first avenue to try. However, most of these activities are very time consuming and you have a baby to look after. So here are three quick and easy ways to relax which you can try out to see which works best for you. Then just use this as often as you can during the day, starting right now. You can do this when you are standing at the sink, feeding baby, hanging out the washing, talking to people, any time really. They are enormously helpful.

1. Scanning

Breathe in while silently scanning your body for any tension.

As you breathe out, relax any tension you found.

Repeat several times.

2. Countdown 1

Focus on your breathing.

Count silently backwards from 10 to 0, saying the next number silently each time you breathe out.

3. Countdown 2

Sit or stand quietly and do a very slow and silent countdown from 10 to 0, and with each downward count, imagine yourself unwinding and letting go a little bit more.

Repeat if necessary.

Q. I do yoga, and they always have a relaxation session at the end. Would that help me with PND?

A. Yes, any sort of relaxation will help you to feel better. If you can do this at home without the yoga teacher talking you through it, that's great. If you can get back out to your yoga class, that's even better.

Easy breathing tips

Breathing is essential for life and is the body's fuel. If we get that very basic of activities wrong, this can upset the whole body chemistry and produce many unexpected symptoms, which you can find yourself worrying about. Light-headedness, tingling in the fingers and toes, poor memory and concentration, panic feelings, and more, can all be brought on by breathing just a little too fast. PND can make you anxious, and anxiety can make you breathe a little bit too fast. So let's make a start to putting that right.

We'll give you more ways of doing this in Chapter 8, but here is one breathing technique to try out now. Don't forget your relaxation exercises though. Try to find time for both. We know this is difficult, but it need only take a few minutes and you may well reap huge benefits. There are always spare minutes in the day which you can use for this if time is a problem – waiting for a bus or a taxi, on the bus or train, queuing at the shops, or while you are feeding the baby.

Try this out first when you are already fairly relaxed until you get a feel for it. Then you can use it regularly throughout each day to keep tension and anxiety at a minimum. You can also use it when you are feeling anxious, to help you to feel better. Sounds simple, but it can be very effective.

1–2–3 Breathing

Lie or sit with good support.

Let your breath go, then take a gentle breath in to your own slow silent count of 1.........2.........3, then breathe out again in your own time to your own slow and silent count of 1.........2.........3.

Continue gently breathing to this rhythm for a minute or two.

MYTH: Taking lots of really deep breaths helps you if you feel anxious or stressed.

FACT: Taking lots of deep breaths will probably make you feel worse. Doing this makes you 'hyperventilate' or 'over breathe'. Slow gentle breathing using tummy muscles rather than upper chest muscles will help you relax.

Q. I'm not good with breathing exercises and the like but I really enjoy walking. I'm out with the pram every day. Will that help me to relax?

A. Yes, provided you enjoy it in the first place, walking is a really good way to unwind and get air into your lungs. Just make sure you walk at a reasonable pace and spend at least 10–15 minutes walking each time.

What is a panic attack?

If you have been having panic attacks, you will be very keen to do something about it. You will know how unpleasant they are, how frightening and how limiting. You will know the difficulties they create and how an attack makes you apprehensive, anxious and fearful of everyday situations. It all sounds miserable and upsetting, but need it be? The point is that you can do something about panic feelings and here is where you start.

When we are anxious or worried, the automatic part of our nervous system becomes aroused. This is the part which keeps us breathing and our heart beating automatically, without our having to think about it. This arousal is a necessary part of our biological make-up and evolved in our cave man ancestors as a self-preservation mechanism, to prepare them to cope *physically* with whatever dangerous situation they might experience.

So, in the case of an approaching snarling sabre-toothed tiger, this instant automatic arousal prepared them to either 'fight' the animal, or 'flee' as fast as they could. This all happens completely automatically, because if our ancestors had taken time to think about it, it would have been too late.

Every split second counted in our early days. We breathe faster, think faster, our heart beats faster, our muscles become taught and ready for action, our blood sugar levels rise to give rapid energy, increased amounts of adrenalin are produced, and so on. All to prepare us for instant and effective action.

Clearly this is a very primitive, but still essential, part of us. If we had to take the time to work out what to do when a speeding car suddenly bears down on us while crossing the street, it would already be too late. The 'fight or flight' reaction does it for us before we have time to think. In terms of evolution, this development was all relatively recent, so our bodies react in exactly the same way today.

However, in our modern world, anxiety and worry is not often caused by *physically* dangerous situations. Your panic feelings are part of your PND, which is making you feel under threat *psychologically*. You don't have to fight or flee from danger, so all those major bodily changes have no outlet, leaving you feeling very strange indeed. This may sound a little complex but it is worth thinking about. After all, what we are describing is a normal physical reaction, something we share with all other animals.

A panic attack like this can be very frightening. It feels like being the victim of a terrifying attack over which you appear to have absolutely no control. You can be convinced that you are going mad or are about to die. So what can you do if you have panic attacks?

How to cope with a panic attack

Once you understand the 'fight or flight' reaction, panic attacks can seem much less frightening. However, from a more practical point of view, you need to learn how to deal with them. If you have panic attacks, the key is to catch them early, and stop them in their tracks. This puts you back in control. Here is one way of doing this but don't be put off if this method doesn't work the first or even second time you try it. Keep at it. It takes a bit of practice and a bit of determination, but it is very effective. Thousands of people have used it successfully. You can too.

The PAUSE routine

First, work out what your own first signs of a panic attack are. This might be a lurch in the stomach, a thought in your mind, your heart rate rising, or something else you've noticed.

Be on the look out for these first signs and, when you notice them, you should immediately:

Pause....and make yourself comfortable (sit down, lean on something etc.)
Absorb....detail of what's going on around you
Use....any method of relaxing quickly which works well for you, *then*
Slowly....when you feel better,
Ease....yourself back into what you were doing.

That's:
P Pause
A Absorb detail around you
U Use relaxation, then
S Slowly,
E Ease yourself back into what you were doing.

This is where the quick ways of relaxing we explained earlier pay off hugely. When using the PAUSE routine, you can use whichever of these methods has worked best for you – be it any of the types of relaxing quickly or the breathing technique.

Coping with angry feelings

Sometimes instead of anxiety or panic, the 'fight or flight' reaction can show itself as anger, and this is quite common in PND. We'll give you more ideas on how to tackle this in Chapter 8, but here are some suggestions which you can try out now:

- Release the anger constructively by doing something physically demanding and useful like hoovering, cleaning, dancing or aerobics.

- Look out for your triggers and, when you are aware of anger beginning, use relaxation or calming breathing of some kind to nip it in the bud, and counteract the feeling.

- If need be, make an excuse and leave the situation for a minute or two. Make sure your baby is safe and secure first. Now, use relaxation and breathing or something else which helps you to calm down like going for a walk or a run, then return when calmer.

- Prevent highs and lows of your blood sugar by avoiding sugary food and eating small and healthy regular meals.

On the spot mood lifters

Here are a few easy and quick ideas for helping to lift your mood when you are feeling down. We will give much more help with this throughout the book, especially in Chapters 8 and 13.

- Put on some cheerful music which you enjoy and has happy associations for you.

- Switch on a light and make sure there's lots of light, natural or otherwise, wherever you go.

- Do something creative – cook, sew, paint, plant some seeds, knit.

- Move around and be active as much as you can.

- Make sure you are eating healthy amounts of protein in your diet every day, for example, lean meat, chicken, fish, milk, nuts, seeds, pulses, eggs and rice, as these can produce mood lifting chemicals.

Having a baby looked so wonderful in all the magazines and I had looked forward to it all so much. The reality couldn't have been more different. Tiredness I could never have imagined, and a never-ending round of nappy, feed, washing, ironing. And I just felt so down all the time and couldn't stop crying. Nobody seemed to understand at all.

Ruth, 17

I had felt truly awful for about three months after my little boy was born, and hadn't told a soul. Then, one day I burst into tears when I was out shopping with a friend, and it all tumbled out. But it was okay. My friend knew exactly what I was talking about. She told me she had felt like that too. I couldn't believe it. That was the day I began to get better.

Alison, 33

Bonding well with your baby

You may be concerned about how all this is affecting the bond with your baby. In Part 2, Chapter 9, we'll give you some help and information about keeping the bond with your baby and any other children strong. Parent–child bonds develop through everyday caring so, in the meantime, make sure you spend as much time as you can with all of your children – soothing them if they are upset, changing nappies, bathing, cuddling, singing and playing with them. You may also want to hold the baby 'skin to skin' – in other words against your own skin whenever you can, and have plenty of eye contact and touching. If it's difficult, start gradually, and build this up a little each day. It doesn't matter that you don't feel much to begin with, this kind of contact will help the bond to form, and help you to fall in love with your baby.

4

How those around
you can help you now

In the first three chapters of Part 1, we explained what baby blues and postnatal depression (PND) are, and gave you some idea of what you should do if you suspect that you have PND. We also gave you some starter self-help tips and thoughts about how your partner and friends might be reacting and how to let them know what has been happening to you, and why. Hopefully, we've also answered some of the main questions and concerns you are likely to have in these very early days. In this last chapter in Part 1, we give you some idea of the many ways that those around you can help you and there is a section for you to give to them to read.

How your partner can help right now

We've already thought about how your partner might be feeling at this time and we've given you some ideas on how you can go about telling him about PND. If he understands what's been happening to you, he can be a tremendous support to you and help you through this very difficult time. When he has had time to come to terms with what is happening to you, it should be easier for him to get involved and help out still more whenever he can. As we said, he may be feeling bad, too, but it is you who is ill, and you who needs maximum support. Do give him some time to take things in and adjust to this new and unknown territory. Let him read the later section in this chapter which will give him lots of ideas to help you and is written for him and for those around you. Do remember that you have to stay active and involved in your life too. You won't get better by sitting back and letting other people do everything, much as it may feel that way. We know it takes a huge effort, but it is worth it, we assure you. We have both been there and we know only too well what it is like.

How your other children can help

When you are already tired, desperately low and disinterested, all the jobs, noise and activity that other children can bring can feel like the last straw. However, when you have PND, having other children around has many positive benefits which you may not have been aware of, and which you can build on and encourage. What benefits can there possibly be, you will be wondering. Well, having others who love and need you will be good for your self-esteem, and this can only help when you are depressed. Then there are the hugs and cuddles, which can help lift a low mood and make you feel wanted. Even though you don't feel like it, and you want to push them away, let them near to you and let them give you their love. They will be feeling insecure as well, so it will be good for them too.

They will also keep you busy. Making meals, organizing homework and sorting out school bags for the next day. Activity of any kind can get those happy chemicals going in your brain and make you feel a little better, so the other children may even have prevented you from feeling much worse.

Your other children will also help to get you out. 'Mummy, you must come to my parents' night. If you don't I'll be the only one whose mummy or daddy didn't come.' Sounds like blackmail, and it is, but giving in to it will do both of you good. Most of the effort involved is in making the decision and actually getting ready to go out. The rest usually falls into place and is much easier and you'll always feel better for going out. Even just dropping your son off at a friend's house, or going to the park to feed the ducks with the pram can make the difference between getting worse and getting better.

The baby's brothers and sisters can also help in other, more practical, ways. They will want to help when they can see that you aren't well, so harness their desire to please you by getting them to give more help around the house. Even the youngest child can do something to help which will take some of the pressure off you, and give you more time to concentrate on doing the things which will make you feel better.

MYTH: Having a good breakfast, lunch and dinner is the best way to eat.

FACT: If it suits you better, you can have five or six smaller meals, especially if you are on the go all the time, or are getting little sleep, or if your appetite is poor.

What family and friends can do

Most people, despite not really understanding and not knowing what to say, will offer practical help. That way, they can at least feel they are doing something for you. You may well be reluctant to accept such offers, as you don't want it to appear that you are not coping. You will probably have been saying 'no' to many people and feeling more useless because they are offering, but you should accept some of these offers. This is not a sign of you not coping or of weakness – you are ill, and people do actually want to help and be involved. It's one of the things they **can** do, especially when they can't find the right words to say. If you had flu or a tummy upset, you wouldn't think twice about accepting help. This is no different. You are ill, just the same. If you are entirely on your own, it is especially important for you to get in touch with one of the support groups we've listed for you in Part 5, so that you can have help like this too.

So, yes, let your mother do the hoovering and your sister a bit of ironing. Maybe a new friend from a local support group can help with the washing. This will help you to keep on top of the housework. If your mum-in-law can pick up some groceries on her way to see you, let her. Even better, accept the babysitting offer she made last week, and have a night out with your partner or some girlfriends. Having more time to yourself and spending time on things which make you feel good is an important part of your road to recovery, so start saying yes, today.

Q. I haven't seen my doctor yet, but I've heard that St John's Wort is good for depression. Should I start taking that now?

A. You'd be better to wait until you have a clear diagnosis of PND and then discuss that with your doctor. This herbal remedy may help with mild to moderate depression, but some herbal remedies can interfere with other medication you are taking and with breastfeeding, so it's best not to try any herbal remedies without medical supervision. There is more on this in Chapter 7.

MYTH: You can't do anything about PND. You just have to put up with it until it goes away.

FACT: There is lots and lots you can do. You don't need to put up with feeling so unhappy and unwell. It's better for those around you too, especially your baby, if you get better as quickly as you can.

Other mums

As we've said already, there will probably be other mums around you, too. Some won't understand PND, but will offer practical help nonetheless. Accept some of these offers. There will also be some mums who have experienced PND for themselves and they will most likely make this known to you somehow. No one understands PND better than another mum who has been through it. It is very common indeed, so you are almost certain to know someone who has been there, and who will be ready and willing to share their experiences with you. A trouble shared really is a trouble halved. It's such a relief not to have to pretend and not to have to put on a happy face. It's so great to be able to really tell someone how it really is, and for them to understand.

Q. Do anti-depressants work straight away?

A. No, depending on the tablet, they may take anything from ten days to a month to work fully. If you are prescribed medication for your PND, ask your doctor, or read the information leaflet which comes with your tablets carefully. There is more on this in Chapter 7.

Support groups

There are many, many great support groups out there, with people who have felt exactly as you do now. They are waiting to share your pain and to take some of your burden from you. There are also national organizations and local groups in most areas. So you can share things with someone nearby, over the phone or face to face, whatever you feel most comfortable with. There are national organizations with email support and email discussion groups, if you prefer a little distance. They all offer lots of useful information about PND developed from many years of personal experience. You can phone or write to them, or you can email them, or visit their website. You may not feel up to this sort of thing yet, but they will still be there when you are ready. You'll find messages from them in Part 4, and a list of contact details in Part 5.

Next steps and Part 2

We've covered a lot in this first part of the book and it's so good that you are still here with us. Well done for that. We know how difficult it can be to concentrate and to make time for yourself. You've taken that first all-important step towards tackling your PND – you've read up to here in this book.

We hope that you've tried out some of the hints and tips we've described for you and that you've found them helpful and they made you feel just a little more relaxed and more positive. Don't worry if you haven't had much benefit yet, as these things can take a bit of time to work. Keep at it and we can assure you that it will be worth it.

In Part 2, we take you on your next steps towards recovery and explain what is happening to you and why. We describe the kinds of treatment you might be offered, including medication, and how these might help. We also answer other concerns you may have and give you lots more practical self-help tips and suggestions of where and how to get emotional and practical support. And don't forget, there is a list of helpful organizations and their contact details in Part 5, if you feel ready to get in touch with someone now.

It's time now to hand over the remainder of this part and this chapter to those around you. The following section is written for them, to give them suggestions on how best to understand what's happening to you, and on how they can help you. You can read it too.

Q. Can I stop taking the medication as soon as I feel better?

A. No, you need to continue with the medication until your doctor feels you can come off the tablets. This may be for a number of months. You must then cut down very gradually, just as you should with most medications you've been taking for some time. There is more on this in Chapter 7.

A message for your partner, friends and family

This section has been specially written for you, to give you some idea how best you can help the woman you know who has postnatal depression (PND). Remember, we know it's been difficult for you too, so if you want more advice or someone to talk to yourself, or you are still worried about anything, don't hesitate to speak to the doctor, midwife or health visitor, or contact one of the helplines or websites given in Part 5. They are not just there to help new mothers, they are there for you too. Here are some other ways that you can help:

- Take PND seriously. It is a real, distressing and serious illness. She isn't lazy, a bad mother, or making anything up.

- Read all of this book.

- Don't tell her she should 'pull herself together'. She will constantly be trying to do this and she just can't. It would be like telling someone to shake themselves out of having flu.

- Make sure she gets regular time for herself. This will help her to feel better more quickly and to cope better with her illness.

- Give her lots and lots of moral support.

- Listen when she wants or needs to talk. This will help her a lot and it will help you to understand things better too.

- Be understanding.

- Don't expect a super tidy house.

- Don't criticize or blame her. None of this is anybody's fault.

- Make sure she is getting enough rest. Let her have naps as often as she needs them.

- Support her decision about how she wants to tackle her PND. Make a point of understanding how PND is treated, especially the treatment she will be having.

- Take her out and about with friends, or just the two of you, without the baby or other children, whenever you can. This will give her (and you) a break and let her feel part of the world again.

- Help out with the housework, without taking over, or appearing to be criticizing her ability to keep the house in order. Ask her how you can help.

- Go with her to appointments if that would help her or you.

- Make sure she is eating properly and regularly. Little and often can sometimes work better than big meals.

- Make sure she is not having to cope alone with the baby too much. This can make her PND worse.

- Collect the other children from school, nursery or playgroup, when you can.

- Help with the children's homework.

- Give the baby a bottle feed at night sometimes, to let her sleep straight through. This will give her a great energy boost. You can even use expressed breast milk for this.

- Help out with the baby.

- Ask often how she is feeling and how you can help and remember to give yourself time to really hear the answer and act on it.

- Be there to support her through the ups and the downs which can inevitably happen on the way to recovery.

- Help her through any more substantial setbacks she may have along the way. Many women have these. This is not her fault and she will come through it with support and understanding.

- Remember to look after yourself too – this isn't easy for you either and you are a very important person.

I had PND about a year ago. My health visitor noticed it very quickly thank goodness. I'm feeling fine now, but at the time it seemed as if my whole world had collapsed around me and I couldn't do anything about it. I had a beautiful healthy baby boy, just what I had wanted, so why wasn't I happy? My mum said it had all been too easy for me and I didn't appreciate how lucky I was. But I did really. I was so hurt by what she said. I just felt I was trapped behind this awful, awful feeling of despair and the panic I felt when I woke up in the morning was terrifying and mind-numbing. I know mum was only trying to help in her own way, but it didn't help at all. I explained this to my health visitor and she told me about a group for new mums, which she organized on a Monday afternoon. I was really scared at first. You hear such stories about women's groups. But it was great. Such a support.

Alisha, 32

Part 2:
Taking Control –
The Early Weeks

5

How the doctor and health visitor can help

In Part 1, we concentrated on immediate reassurance and explanation for you, and we had a kind of 'first aid' approach to postnatal depression (PND). In this second part of the book, we take you on your next tentative steps and help you through the first weeks of working towards your recovery. In other words, your first moves towards regaining control of your life. We will explain in greater detail what is happening to you and why, because just understanding why you feel the way you do can make a tremendous difference and lift some of that huge weight off your shoulders. It can also help you to understand that you have nothing at all to be ashamed of or to feel guilty about. You wouldn't feel ashamed if you had a torn muscle, a cold or a kidney infection, so you shouldn't feel ashamed if you have PND. There is no difference.

This chapter focuses on how the doctor or health visitor can help you. Chapter 6 will then explain what we know about the causes of PND. Then, with a better understanding of the causes, in Chapter 7, we will discuss the kinds of treatment you might be offered. We will help you to decide which treatment you want, if any, by telling you how these might help and how long you might expect it to take until you really feel better. We will also address any concerns you may have about breastfeeding while on medication. There will be plenty of practical self-help tips in Chapter 8, and many suggestions of where to get emotional and practical support, including from other mothers experiencing PND. Chapter 9 will explain the kind of pattern of recovery you can expect in these early weeks and also give you ideas on how to strengthen the bond with your baby and your other children.

First steps – making an appointment

If you think there is any chance at all that you might have PND, you should make an appointment with your doctor straight away. Do it today. Do it now. The doctor won't mind at all if it turns out you don't have PND. Doctors would much rather you came to see them to get it checked out, than sat at home wondering what to do. They will soon decide one way or another. As we've said already, if you have any thoughts at all about harming yourself, or harming the baby, call the doctor straight away and tell the person who answers the call how you are feeling. They won't be shocked and they will be able to help you. Don't worry about phoning out of hours – all areas have a full out-of-hours service these days and the medical staff are waiting to help you. There is no point in risking your safety or your baby's. If your best friend were feeling the way you are, what would you advise them to do?

Q. I am only slightly down. Should I still see a doctor?

A. It's probably always worth seeing the doctor, as your 'slightly down' may be someone else's 'very depressed'. If the doctor feels that you can cope without treatment, there are lots of self-help ideas in Chapter 8.

What to tell the doctor

There are three main areas to discuss with your doctor – your feelings, your behaviour and your thinking. Tell him or her how you are feeling, physically and emotionally. Explain any of your behaviour that worries you and tell the doctor about any of your thoughts which you are unhappy about. We realize that you might find this difficult and that before you had the baby you would have been able to explain how you were feeling without any problem, but just at the moment you may find it awkward.

You are probably feeling really low or just have no confidence in yourself right now. You may find doctors intimidating and a symbol of authority and you might be a bit in awe of them or even scared of them. You might want to call one of the helplines given in Part 5 first, if you feel that would help build your confidence.

Take someone with you if you feel you need that familiar support, even if it's just to keep you company in the waiting room. It's sometimes good to take someone with you, who knows you well anyway, because they can sometimes explain even better than you can just what you have been going through and how you have changed since the baby was born. They may well have noticed differences in you that you haven't been aware of yourself.

If you find it easier to talk to a woman, make an appointment with a female doctor. You can see any doctor in most practices these days, not just the one you're registered with. Don't worry – your own doctor won't be at all offended by this. If you feel that you'll forget what you want to say, write it down and hand it to the doctor or ask your partner, mother or best friend to go in with you and explain things for you. Lack of confidence and anxieties like these can all be part of the PND. Having PND can make even everyday behaviour, which you used to take for granted, seem so very difficult and such an enormous mountain to climb.

Do remember that doctors are just people, like you; people who have just learned a bit more about the body and how it works. They are the same as you and me, and they are there to help. They want to help you. It's their job to help you, so don't feel at all guilty about 'bothering' them. You have an illness and you need help with it.

How the doctor can help you

The doctor will probably ask you some questions about how you have been feeling and behaving, and the diagnosis of PND will be based on what you tell him or her and the kinds of symptoms you've been having. There isn't a blood or urine test which will come up red or green, or with a line, if you have PND. Things would probably be a lot easier if there was such a test. You may be given a straightforward questionnaire to fill in, or the doctor may ask you the questions from it, and this will tell the doctor much more about whether you have PND and how severe it is. A commonly used questionnaire is the 'Edinburgh Postnatal Depression Scale', which has ten questions, but a range of these scales is now used throughout the UK to screen for PND in new mums.

MYTH: If I go to the doctor about feeling down after the baby, she'll send me to see a psychiatrist.

FACT: That would be extremely unusual for PND. Even if you did see a psychiatrist, that would be because the doctor thought they could help you best. Psychiatrists are experts on PND and on its treatment. Everything would be confidential too.

That said, the doctor may ask you to take some other medical tests, just to make sure you don't also have an underlying physical problem, which can produce some of the same symptoms as PND and is quite common in new mothers. So he or she may, for example, ask you for a blood sample to test if you're anaemic or have an under-active thyroid or you may be asked to bring in a sample of urine so that you can be checked for diabetes. All of these conditions can produce some of the same symptoms as PND.

If the doctor decides you have PND, the various treatment options will then be explained to you. You may be given some leaflets to read on the subject. The doctor may ask you to make another appointment, when the treatment options will be explained, because you may not be able to take much in at a first appointment. In Chapter 7, we will explain these various options in detail for you.

Q. Does having PND mean that I am mentally ill?

A. No, it doesn't. PND is usually thought of as a 'psychological problem' or 'psychological disorder'.

How the health visitor or midwife can help you

If you prefer to talk to your midwife, as you have got to know her, or to your health visitor, then just make an appointment with them or give them a call. The system will vary in different parts of the UK, but you should have information about what to do to contact help of that kind. If not, just call your doctor's practice and they will give you the contact numbers. All health professionals will be very understanding and completely unshockable, so don't be afraid to explain things to them and ask about anything at all which is worrying you. It is quite likely that they will come out to visit you at home, rather than you having to go in to the surgery with the baby, or having to organize a babysitter.

The health visitor can also check if you have PND by talking with you and using the same sort of questionnaire as a doctor would. They may also explain about the various treatment options available to you and answer any of your questions. They will probably ask you to make an appointment with your doctor if you have PND, so that he or she can organize any treatment you decide on.

Even if the health visitor isn't the first person you contact about PND, they are likely to provide you with ongoing support while you are recovering. They will visit you at home and you can talk to them about any concerns you have about yourself or about the baby. They can even help you to cope with your baby's sleeping problems, feeding difficulties or nappy rash and can introduce you to local mother's groups or breastfeeding groups.

MYTH: If I tell the midwife or the health visitor how I feel, they'll just think I'm a useless mother.

FACT: Nobody will think that. All health professionals understand PND and know it's not your fault. They will be on your side. You must be honest about this, so that you can get help.

Everybody kept telling me how well I was coping and how beautiful Jamie was. And yet, behind closed doors, it was all so very different. I just kept asking myself why I couldn't tell them what was really going on, and how I was really feeling.

Corinne, 30

I had the usual baby blues after my two daughters, but it was nothing compared to the depression I had after the birth of my son. I cried constantly and didn't want to know my kids, husband or friends. I wasn't sleeping and was completely obsessed by housework. My husband eventually phoned the doctor, and a health visitor came out to see me. I was so angry with him. I can barely even remember that day, it is just a blur now, but thank goodness my husband did what he did.

Philippa, 42

6

What causes PND?

We will now take a bit of time out to explain some of the current thinking about what causes postnatal depression (PND). Some mothers are really interested in knowing about this and keep asking themselves why this has happened to them. Others may not be at all bothered about why they have PND and may just want to know how they are going to get better. Whichever way you feel about this, we would strongly encourage you to read through this chapter because understanding the cause can sometimes help you to feel a little better and knowing something about the causes of PND will mean that the treatments will make a lot more sense when we come to explain them in Chapter 7.

The causes of PND

It is not known for certain what causes PND, but it seems likely that in some cases it is the sudden change in hormones after the birth which may be the trigger. Some people think of this as a complication of pregnancy. There has been a lot of research into the causes of PND and this has shown that a number of factors may be involved, rather than just one direct and obvious reason. A number of different possibilities has been put forward to explain why new mothers may become depressed in this way and any one of these, or a combination of them, can be contributing to your PND.

Whatever the cause, the outcome is thought to be an imbalance in the chemical messengers in your brain, in particular, levels of a messenger called 'serotonin'. This chemical messenger is particularly involved in setting your mood and anxiety levels.

So, apart from the hormonal changes, what other factors might be causing your PND?

Stress of a new baby

The first of these factors is stress. Depression at other times is often caused by emotional and stressful events and although we know that having a baby is usually a joyous and welcome event, it is nonetheless also a very stressful one. Having a baby involves many changes in your body, your life and your lifestyle, and change is known to be very stressful. Other stressful events around the birth can also make PND more likely.

MYTH: Babies are always clean, beautifully dressed and smiling, as they appear to be in most adverts.

FACT: Babies are like that a lot of the time, and this is wonderful, but they can also be fretful, cry, and be very messy and demanding.

Any of the points in the following checklist can produce stress during pregnancy and after the birth, and so encourage the development of depression. Do any of these apply to you? Tick any that do. The more that apply, the more stress you were experiencing:

❑ A difficult delivery.

❑ Not much help and support at home.

❑ No close family or friends nearby.

❑ Physical health problems, such as urinary difficulties, anaemia, or wound infections, following the birth.

❑ Your baby had health problems.

❑ Your baby cried a lot or was very unsettled or colicky.

❑ Your baby had feeding difficulties.

❑ Frequent breastfeeding on demand.

It is worth pointing out that your baby's delivery may have been perfectly normal and routine, but you found it difficult, embarrassing and traumatic because it just wasn't what you were expecting. How can you really know what to expect? It's completely new territory for every woman. Films and television can depict a birth as a quick and simple event, which doesn't even disturb your hair or make-up, and involves no mess and relatively little pain. There can also be a bit of a conspiracy of silence around the realities of childbirth. Other mothers often keep quiet about the realities of it, so as not to discourage you. Though to be fair on other mothers, you do forget any pain and discomfort very quickly after the birth.

MYTH: A bit of stress is good for you.

FACT: No amount of stress is good for you. If you are feeling stressed or anxious, then you are feeling you can't cope with something. That's not good for you. A bit of challenge or excitement in your life can be good for you, but not stress.

Unrealistic expectations about motherhood

As if all this wasn't enough, it may be that having unrealistic expectations about being a mother can also contribute strongly to developing PND. Once again, this isn't your fault. Magazines, television programmes, advertising and films are full of marvellous images of how wonderful it is to be a mother, and are full of images of happy, gurgling, smiling and beautifully clean babies. Of course this is part of the truth – babies are magical, gorgeous and mind-blowing little beings, and becoming a mother is the most extraordinarily wonderful experience you could ever imagine – but there is so much more to it than that.

There is the loss of freedom and the relentlessness of a baby's needs. The feeding and changing routine, which was a novelty at first, can soon feel like a ball and chain, especially if you are breastfeeding on demand. There is the constant messiness and smelliness, your clothes and hair always smell of sick, or worse. Sometimes, the joy of at last being a mother is simply lost in a sea of pain, stretch marks, incredibly dirty nappies, and trying to get the baby to 'fix' to your breast for a feed, or wind him after his bottle.

Loss

A common reason for depression at any time in your life is a loss of some kind. Loss of a job, a loved one, a relationship, financial loss or a dear pet dying. Becoming a mother involves many losses, not only of freedom, but also of income, of independence and of your sense of who you are. Your appearance will have changed from your old familiar figure and nowadays you won't have time for make-up, choosing what to wear and all of that. But all that was part of what made you feel like you. Your old relationship with your partner may well have gone too. It is common for a new mother to be less interested in sex, and then there is a new person in the house to spend time on. Going out socially becomes a major planning exercise, when it used only to need a second's decision time. All the old exciting spontaneity has gone. Your social life with your friends and with your partner will suffer too. So much of what was familiar and comforting for you may well have disappeared. You can feel lost and not a little bewildered – and you're not really sure why. It can all make you feel so ungrateful, and so very, very, guilty and ashamed.

The shock of the responsibility

Then of course there is the sudden and complete responsibility of it all. Suddenly being responsible for another tiny human being can come as quite a shock, even though you knew it was going to happen. You are responsible for this tiny crying child 24 hours a day, and it is so very difficult to know what is wrong when they cry. The books you read make it all sound so straightforward, but the more anxious you become about the crying, the more the baby cries, sensing your insecurity and tension as you hold him. This can feel quite overwhelming, especially if you've had no experience of babies or children before. You can find yourself losing even more sleep, because you lie awake listening for the baby breathing, terrified of cot death.

Then there is the desperate and all-consuming tiredness that only a new baby in the house can bring. If you have never had a broken night's sleep before, you will find even one a major shock to your system. But one, followed by another, and still another, with no let-up, is so very exhausting. Life can become dominated by the ever growing mound of washing and ironing and visitors trooping in to 'see the baby'. 'What about me?' you find yourself asking. Aren't they here to see me too?

You have become invisible. You have joined that invisible army of mothers who trudge along day after day, looking after the needs of other people. This can also come as a terrific shock. We can assure you that the shock does subside, and you will become used to it, and you will even come to enjoy motherhood. However, the shock can show itself as PND, because you don't have an opportunity to show it any other way. You're supposed to be over the moon. You're supposed to be elated, fulfilled and glowing, as all new mothers are. So you keep your feelings to yourself.

Q. I didn't stop work until very near to the birth. Could that have caused my PND?

A. Provided you were feeling fit and well, weren't too tired and were well prepared for the baby coming, it shouldn't make any difference when you left work.

Adjusting

Another possibility in the UK is that a birth is not marked in any way, as is the case for a wedding or a death. Rituals like weddings and funerals are sometimes called 'rites of passage', and these help us to adjust to a new role in our lives. The organization MIND gives an example from India, where a new mother might spend the first six weeks mainly in bed with the baby, with the women of the family around her, helping, singing and telling stories. Customs like this allow the new mother to recover from the birth and get to know her new baby. She also has a chance to learn mothering skills from other women in the family. Even in the UK, just 20 years ago, new mothers could spend a week in hospital recovering, resting and learning how to feed and care for their babies.

Isolation

When you have been used to going out to work every day and socializing with friends and family whenever you felt like it, being at home on your own with a new baby can feel like a very isolating experience. Even if you have your mum and friends dropping by, there will still be long stretches of the day where it's just you and the baby, and babies are not the most communicative of creatures for the first few months. You have to wait at least a month for a quick smile and a proper conversation is out of the question for a long time yet.

Neighbourhoods are much less close-knit these days, so you may not even know who your neighbours are, let alone have a chat over the fence or drop round for a morning coffee. That's if your neighbours are in during the day at all. In the winter especially, with very short days, neighbours can leave before your blinds are open and return after they are closed. If you live in a high rise flat, or anonymous housing estate, you can feel particularly isolated from the world. This will probably be the first time this has happened to you, so it can be especially hard to take, especially if you are a very social person and not at all used to your own company.

What has caused your PND?

Did you identify with anything in this chapter? Has it given you a better idea of what may have contributed to your PND? As we said at the beginning of the chapter, it can help quite a lot just to know why you are suffering in this awful way when you should be happy, relaxed and fulfilled. It can also make understanding and choosing a treatment plan much more straightforward for you, as we will see in the next chapter.

Q. I had a glass or two of wine most weeks while I was pregnant. Could that be why I have PND?

A. There is no definite evidence one way or another about this, but it is very unlikely. However, you are probably better to avoid alcohol completely if you become pregnant again, as we don't really know how this might affect you or your baby.

*I had wanted a baby for years. Ever
since I played with my dolls when I was
little, I wanted a real one to look after
and love. My wedding was a dream and
then I became pregnant really easily.
Now I just look at her and I can't feel
any connection. I don't feel that 'wow'
feeling I expected. Worst of all, I just
feel so ashamed. How can I feel this
way when I have everything I ever
wanted?*

Geeta, 33

7

Treatment options

We hope that the last chapter about the causes of postnatal depression (PND) was useful. It can help such a lot when you have a better understanding of a condition like PND. It can feel really frightening not knowing what's going on, and that just makes your anxiety and depression worse. So now you understand PND a little better, what is your next step? The most likely thing that you will be doing now is getting in touch with your doctor or the health visitor. This chapter will describe the sorts of treatment that they may offer to you if they confirm that you have PND.

How is PND treated?

If you had a chest infection, measles or a broken arm, things would be straightforward, with just one way of treating the condition. Things are not so simple with PND, there isn't only one option. Just as we were saying in Chapter 6 about the causes of PND being many and varied, the same is true of its treatment. Though there may be a number of different alternatives, be assured that they are all very effective. You are an individual after all, so you have to find the treatment which best suits you and your needs.

There may be a little trial and error involved in selecting the best option for you, but you could think of this as being like getting the right size and style of new outfit for a special event. You may have to try on a few before you find the right one. With your doctor's and health visitor's help you will very quickly arrive at the best treatment for you.

What is more, you **will** have a say in the matter. If you have PND, nothing will be forced upon you. You should be able to choose and you should be able to take some time to make a decision if you need it. You can talk things over with your partner or your family or friends before deciding. You will also be able to change your mind. Being indecisive is often a part of PND. So, what sort of help is available for you to choose from?

Medication

We'll start with the treatment you have probably heard most about already, medication. According to the Royal College of Psychiatrists (RCP) in the UK, there are almost 30 different kinds of antidepressants available today. No one is really sure, but it is thought that antidepressants work by increasing the activity of certain chemicals in our brains called neurotransmitters. We told you a bit about these in Chapter 6. These chemicals pass signals from one brain cell to another. The chemicals most involved in depression are thought to be serotonin, which we've mentioned already, and also noradrenaline. The antidepressants developed some years ago are just as effective as the more recent ones but, on the whole, the newer

---

MYTH: I'm weak if I have to take pills for PND.

FACT: You would take pills for a headache, high blood pressure or a urine infection. PND is no different. It is an illness just the same. So it is not weak to take pills, it is normal and sensible.

ones seem to have fewer side effects.

There are four main types, from the oldest, called 'Tricyclics' to the most recent 'SNRIs'. These are:

- Tricyclics

- MAOIs (Monoamine Oxidase Inhibitors)

- SSRIs (Selective Serotonin Reuptake Inhibitors)

- SNRIs (Serotonin and Noradrenaline Reuptake Inhibitors)

You'll need to be prepared to wait a week or two for any of these pills to work as they don't work straight away. Most people find that they take between one and two weeks to start working and maybe up to six weeks to give their full effect. Do stick with it. It is also very important to take them every day, as this is how they are designed to do you the most good. Don't be tempted to stop taking them as soon as you are feeling a little better – giving up your antidepressants too early is the commonest reason for not recovering and for PND returning.

MYTH: Antidepressants are addictive.

FACT: Antidepressants aren't addictive in the way alcohol or smoking is, but you may feel some effects when you come off them, especially if you stop them suddenly. These effects should only be temporary though, and are reduced by cutting down gradually.

Q. Will I have to go into hospital?

A. It is extremely unlikely if you are suffering from PND. You would only be admitted to hospital in the severest of cases, or if you have another form of postnatal illness called 'postnatal psychosis' (see Chapter 12) – and in some cases you can take your baby with you, into a special mother and baby unit.

I'm worried about taking tablets

You may not like the idea of taking tablets. You will not be alone in feeling like that. We can assure you now that medication for depression is very helpful for most people. But after thinking it through carefully, if you are still absolutely sure that you don't want to take tablets, talk this over with your doctor. There are other treatments you can try and we'll explain these shortly. No one will force you to take medication if you really don't want to.

Side effects from medication

All medications have side effects and anti-depressants are no different. The most common side effects are a dry mouth and a bit of nausea or indigestion. The earlier, older medications may also make you sleepy and slow down your reactions. Make sure to read the leaflet which comes with your medication thoroughly and always remind the doctor of any other conditions you have as this may be relevant.

Try not to be put off if you get some side effects at the start. Most of them wear off in a few days. This is just your body adjusting to the new medication. Stick with it, and don't stop the tablets unless the side effects really are unpleasant. If they are, get an urgent appointment to see your doctor. If you feel worse instead of better, it is important to tell your doctor straight away so that they can decide if the medicines are right for you. Your doctor will also want to know if you get increased feelings of restlessness or agitation, or feel more depressed. If you find a particular medication isn't helping, don't give up and put up with your PND. It is very common and if you tell your doctor, they can prescribe another one which may work better for you.

Are antidepressants addictive?

Another reason that many people are concerned about taking tablets is the worry about becoming addicted or dependent on them. According to the RCP, antidepressants don't cause the addictions that you get with tranquillizers, alcohol or cigarettes. What can happen is that when you stop taking your medication, especially if you stop suddenly, you can have what are known as withdrawal symptoms. Most medication that you've been taking for some time will have some withdrawal effects when you stop taking it. These are caused by your body readjusting itself.

The RCP says that up to a third of people who stop SSRIs and SNRIs can have withdrawal symptoms, so you might have a bit of a stomach upset, flu-like symptoms or dizziness. Some people can feel a bit anxious again, but this is not the PND coming back and should pass. You might also have some vivid dreams and strange feelings for a while. It is always best to gradually reduce your medication over a period of weeks or months, rather than just stopping overnight. If you experience anything which concerns you, have a word with your doctor. There is much more on this in Chapter 10.

Taking medication while breastfeeding

Some antidepressants do come through in breastmilk, but be assured, the amounts are very small and are unlikely to cause any harm to the baby. Some antidepressants are better than others in this regard and it is worth talking to your doctor about this. She is likely to choose a drug that is well established and has a good safety record with breastfeeding mothers rather than a newer drug with less evidence about confirming its safety in babies.

> *Q. Is there any difference between PND and the kind of depression I might have at other times?*
>
> **A.** There is some disagreement about this, but many professionals agree that they are very similar, if not the same thing. The symptoms are certainly very alike.

'Talking' treatments

It can be a great relief just to talk to a sympathetic, understanding and uncritical listener. This needn't be a professional, it could just as easily be a good and trusted friend or relative. This can be all some women need. Many doctor's surgeries now have a specially trained counsellor, psychotherapist or health visitor who can help to treat PND. Alternatively, this could be available in a local community based clinic. You are extremely unlikely to be referred to a psychiatrist.

These so-called 'talking therapies' can be really helpful in treating PND. So you may be offered support such as psychotherapy or Cognitive Behavioural Therapy (CBT), which in their different ways offer you the opportunity to look at the underlying factors that have contributed to the PND, as well as helping you to change the way you are feeling and behaving. Psychotherapy can especially help you to understand the depression in terms of what has happened to you in the past. CBT can help you to understand and resolve the depression by examining how you think in the here and now, about yourself, the world and other people.

What is psychotherapy?

There are many different types of psychotherapy. They are all ways of helping people to overcome emotional problems, relationship problems or troublesome habits. What they have in common is that they are all treatments based on talking to another person who has been specially trained. Psychodynamic psychotherapy focuses on the feelings we have about other people, especially our family and those we are close to. Treatment involves discussing past experiences and how these may have led to your present situation and also how these past experiences may be affecting your life now. The understanding gained frees you to make choices about what happens in the future.

What is Cognitive Behaviour Therapy (CBT)?

CBT is another form of talking therapy which is being used more and more often these days to treat different types of depression, including PND. You would be referred to see a specialist therapist, who might be a specially trained nurse, counsellor, psychologist or doctor. They would explain what CBT is all about, and see you for perhaps six to ten sessions of 30–60 minutes. CBT is a way of talking about how you think about yourself, the world and other people; how what you do affects your thoughts and feelings; and how your thoughts can affect your behaviour and your mood.

CBT can help you to change how you think ('cognitive') and what you do ('behaviour'). These changes can help you to feel better. Unlike some of the other talking treatments, it focuses on the 'here and now' problems and difficulties. Instead of focusing on the causes of your distress or symptoms in the past, it looks for ways to improve your state of mind now. CBT can help you to break this vicious circle of altered thinking, feelings and behaviour.

Hormone treatment

If you have had PND before, your doctor may suggest using the hormone progesterone as a way of preventing this happening again. This is given by injection immediately after your baby is born and then later in gradually smaller amounts. You then need to use progesterone pessaries until your periods start again. This is a fairly new treatment, but early signs are that it can be helpful. Your doctor should be able to give you more information about this.

Complementary therapies

Many women have found therapies such as reflexology, relaxation of all kinds, massage, aromatherapy and so on of some benefit. These are holistic therapies, acting on the whole person to support and relax them, rather than intervening in a chemical way. You'll find simple relaxation exercises to try in Chapters 3 and 8 of this book. If you find these particularly effective, you may like to take them further and look into this type of therapy. As the name suggests, these therapies can complement, rather than replace, conventional treatment so, for example, there's no reason why you can't have some aromatherapy sessions at the same time as taking antidepressants or attending sessions of CBT. There is no evidence, however, that complementary therapies alone will effectively treat PND.

Herbal remedies

You will doubtless have seen the vast array of herbal remedies in the shops these days and might wonder if these could work for you. Maybe you've tried some of these already. Individual reactions to these therapies vary, so if you want to try any of these, it is important to talk this over with your doctor. If you want to try a herbal remedy, remember that they can still be very powerful even if they come from plants. 'Natural' doesn't always mean safe and remedies such as St John's Wort can interfere with the effects of other medications you are taking and is not recommended at all if you are breastfeeding. It's best to check with your doctor before trying any of these out.

Talking or tablets?

This can very much depend on where you live and on your doctor's preferences. You may be offered both or you may be offered just one of these options. Talking therapies are thinner on the ground as they are more expensive and more labour intensive than medication. There may be quite a long waiting list for a 'talking treatment' too. Antidepressants and talking treatments are both effective, but antidepressants are perhaps more likely to be recommended if the depression is severe or has gone on for a long time. They can also work a little more quickly than talking treatments.

Your doctor or health visitor will be willing to give advice. It is also sometimes helpful to talk over the options with your family or a close friend. It is important that you feel comfortable with the choice of help or treatment.

Treating PND is not yet an exact science, as we've said already, so you may need to do a bit of trying things out, and it does vary from person to person. What's right for your friend may not work for you at all. There's no real way of predicting. So don't be downhearted if the first thing you try doesn't have much effect. Keep trying. You'll hit the right solution soon enough.

What if you don't want treatment?

Many mothers with PND don't realize what's happening to them or their PND is very mild and they don't come forward for help. Others are too ashamed and keep it a secret, so they are not diagnosed with PND and simply struggle on. Most women like this will actually get better without any treatment after a period of months or sometimes longer. You can get through PND without treatment. However, this can mean a lot of unnecessary suffering and may even lead to bouts of depression recurring later on. Also, PND may completely spoil the experience of being a new mother and put a strain on your relationship with your baby and your partner. So the shorter it lasts, the better. It's important to get help as soon as possible to relieve the depression and to support your developing relationship with your baby. This will help your baby's development in the long run, and sustain your relationship with your partner and other members of the family. It is also likely to be best for your health in the longer term.

Other forms of postnatal illness

There is a very rare, but severe, form of depression which can also occur after giving birth. This is called 'postnatal psychosis' and develops in about one in 1,000 mothers. Some of the symptoms include irrational behaviour and confusion, as well as the symptoms of depression, including suicidal thoughts. Mothers who are affected may also have hallucinations, irrational thoughts and delusions, and often have no idea at all that they are ill. Postnatal psychosis is a serious mental illness. It is very important to see your doctor if you, or a close family member or friend, are at all worried about this. Women with postnatal psychosis are likely to need immediate specialist psychiatric treatment. More on this in Part 3, Chapter 12.

Q. Can you get depressed before the baby is born?

A. Yes. It's important to know that depression can occur during pregnancy as well. This is more common than you might think and can be helped in much the same way as postnatal depression.

I have three children, the oldest is 17, the youngest is 11 now. I've had depression off and on since my eldest was born. I was given pills at the time, but they didn't seem to be working, so I stopped taking them. It was the same with both of my other children and I was depressed, tearful and lacking in confidence after each one. I thought that the pills didn't work for me, so I just got on with things. Life was pretty miserable and my husband just wasn't interested. I've been depressed off and on now for the past 17 years, since Cheryl, my eldest, was born. Then, a few months ago, I thought it was worth another try so I went to the doctor. He prescribed antidepressants and told me I had to be patient this time and keep on taking the tablets. I did and they have made such a difference, I can't begin to tell you. It's like seeing the world through a new pair of eyes.

Sally, 46

8

How you can help yourself

There is a lot of treatment available from your doctor but whether or not you decide to go for treatments like antidepressants or 'talking therapy', there is still so much you can do straight away to help yourself. We've given you little tasters throughout the book so far, but in this chapter we will focus entirely on a variety of straightforward things you can do now, and in the coming weeks and months, to help yourself.

One step at a time

Don't try to do everything all at once. Trying to do too many new things all at once will only make you feel more tired and agitated, so concentrate on just one thing at a time. Step by step is the surest way to make and maintain good progress and, as is often said, the longest of journeys begin with a single step. You can always refer back to this chapter regularly for more ideas once you've mastered a few main changes. Where are you going to start? Keep this at the back of your mind as you read on. You can tick or highlight any of the suggestions that appeal to you.

Relaxation

Back in Chapter 3, we gave you some quick ways to relax and some really effective breathing techniques. We do hope that you've managed to try these out and that they have been helping you to relax. We also explained what to do if you have panic attacks. Here is a method which eases you more slowly into relaxing and which lasts a bit longer. First an important message before you try this out for yourself.

Take care!

The techniques given in this chapter will help you to relax, but they may also reduce your alertness and even make you feel drowsy. While you're working on these and for around ten minutes afterwards, you shouldn't be driving, looking after the baby, or operating machinery, and you shouldn't stand up suddenly.

Tense then relax – total relaxation

Now it's time to try out tensing and relaxing your muscles, to help your body to relax. If you are in any doubt about your physical fitness to try this, check with your doctor. If you still have a wound which is not completely healed, then don't tense that area. If you have raised blood pressure, it is probably better not to try this activity. Stick with the methods in Chapter 3. Here is what to do.

- Lie or sit comfortably, head supported if possible.
- Deliberately make a fist and tense up both hands really hard for five or six seconds...hold it...now let the tension go.

- Slowly repeat this for each of the following parts of your body in turn:

  arms
  shoulders
  neck and head
  face
  back and chest
  tummy and bottom
  legs, feet and toes.

- Relax for a few minutes, and enjoy.

- Rouse yourself gradually.

Q. Recovering from PND seems to take a long time. It's the 21st century, why isn't there a fast, easy cure?

A. It's very frustrating, but there are some illnesses that take a bit longer to get over, and unfortunately PND is one of these. But medicine is progressing all the time, and hopefully faster treatments will be developed soon.

Relaxing your mind

The best way to take your mind off your worries is to give it something else to think about, and the way to make it relax is to give it something relaxing to think about. So let's give this a try. Find a quiet place, where you're not going to be disturbed, try this out and see what works best for you:

- Slow down and relax your body using one of the methods from Chapter 3, or the 'total relaxation' earlier in this chapter.

- Once relaxed, picture as clearly as you can or focus your mind entirely on any one of these for a few minutes:

  – waves lapping on the seashore
  – branches swaying in the breeze
  – deep dark green velvet
  – a word or phrase such as peace, calm, relax
  – a calming poem, prayer or picture.

How you can improve your thinking

When your mood is low, this will often mean that your thinking can become very negative. It can even sometimes be obsessive or a little paranoid. You may have a running commentary in your head, saying, 'I'm useless, I can't do this, I'm going to make a fool of myself, they'll think I'm useless', and so on. Don't worry, this is all part of being depressed. Just being aware of some of the ways that thinking can contribute to depression can make a real difference, and once you are aware of it, you're half-way to changing it. Here are some self-help ideas to try:

Self-help ideas

- Don't ignore the ordinary or good things that happen each day as if they don't count for some reason. Take account of the bad side of life but don't dwell on it.

- When things go wrong it's not always your fault. Other people or the situation are just as often to blame.

- Take your mind off your problems as much as you can. They grow bigger the more you concentrate on them.

- Do you often find yourself using one of these words, 'I **must** do this', 'I **ought** to do that', and so on? Ask yourself who is setting these personal standards and targets and whether you are setting them too high. Let yourself off the hook and lower these standards if necessary.

- If you have worrying or obsessive thoughts that you can't get out of your mind, try thinking (or saying out loud) the word 'STOP!' slowly over and over until your mind goes onto something else. It takes practice, but it can really help. Try it out first when you don't really need it. You'll find you'll get better at it the more you do it. You can use any word or phrase for this which suits you, for example, **stop, calm my mind, leave my mind, go away now, I don't want you in my mind, disappear now**.

- Another way to get rid of unwanted thoughts is to try any mental activity that requires concentration, such as counting backwards from 100 in sevens; repeating a times table; trying to think of a boy's or girl's name for every letter of the alphabet or an animal or a food.

- If you're thinking people are against you, or someone has done something to offend you, or that you can't do something, challenge your thoughts with questions such as: Who says? Where is the evidence for this? Is there another explanation? What would I say to a friend in the same position?

Take regular breaks

When you have a family to think about, having a break may be the last thing on your mind. However, if you want to feel well, and stay well, having regular breaks is essential. Call it 'me-time', 'quality time' or 'work/life balance', it all comes down to the same thing. You need to have time for yourself. So take regular breaks, every day, and every week. A weekend away, alone with your partner, can work wonders.

Even a ten-minute break in a hectic morning to read a magazine and have a fruit juice can be so refreshing. You can do this when the baby is sleeping. Give yourself little treats too. No need for them to be expensive. A lazy bubbly bath or your favourite fruit tea can lift your mood. Make time for yourself and for hobbies, interests and leisure pursuits. This takes your mind off your troubles and helps to keep them in perspective. It also gives your tired body and nervous system a well-deserved break. The housework can wait ten minutes – you can't.

Helping with mood swings

One of the main reasons people get grumpy or angry, seemingly out of the blue, is because their blood sugar level is low. Low blood sugar can make you more likely to feel bad-tempered or angry, and this can happen if you haven't eaten for some time. To avoid highs and lows of your blood sugar, you should eat small and healthy regular meals and avoid refined sugar products. Have a healthy snack between meals, too. So no skipping breakfast and then filling up on a chocolate bar or chocolate biscuit for elevenses. This will just give you a high, followed by a sudden dip, and that's the danger time for a black mood or a bout of aggression and negative thinking.

How exercise can help

Not only is exercise good for elevating your mood as we've seen already, but physical activity has a releasing effect on tension. Exercise can even allow you to use up feelings of anger and frustration safely and usefully. The key is to find a regular activity which you enjoy and which fits in easily with your lifestyle. Getting out for a daily walk with your baby is an easy way to do this. You should of course always check with your doctor if you're unsure about your fitness to begin or resume any exercise or activity routine – though walking is generally okay for most people.

What to do if you are angry

We gave you some help with this in Chapter 3, and our advice above about mood swings can also help to keep anger from rising. On page 156 are some other suggestions you may find helpful for when you feel anger welling up.

Q. Why can't I stop worrying and having these negative thoughts all the time?

A. What you're thinking seems like something you should be able to change at will. But thoughts like these can be more persistent than we expect. Relaxing both your mind and body completely and focusing on positive thoughts and images can be really effective. Meditation also makes this less of a problem for you.

Dealing with anger

- Look out for your triggers and, when you are aware of anger beginning, use relaxation or calming breathing of some kind to 'nip it in the bud', counteract the feeling and relax your tense muscles.

- If need be, make an excuse and leave the situation for a minute or two, allow yourself to calm down, and return when calmer. Make sure the baby is safe first.

- Try not to use angry words – explain and talk about what your feelings are and why.

- Try to keep your voice relaxed and low-key.

- Replace angry thoughts with calming images, for example, a beach, quiet brook, your anger as a fire inside you being 'put out' by a bucket of water.

- Don't mind-read other people's thoughts and intentions – you'll normally be wrong.

How to be more assertive

Everyone's behaviour will vary from situation to situation, but if a lot of what we do is not assertive, this can cause anxiety, mood swings and stress. Being assertive whenever you can is also another way to cope with anger and frustration. Many people think that being assertive means being aggressive and self-centred but this isn't what being assertive is all about. Assertiveness is based around these four ideas:

- Having respect for yourself and others.

- Every human being having equal rights.

- Knowing and expressing your needs.

- Being able to compromise with others.

Instead of being assertive, you may find yourself being manipulative, aggressive or passively giving in all the time. If this is you, here are some ways to become more assertive:

How to say 'No'

- Keep it short and say it confidently and warmly.

- Only give a reason if you want to.

- Use a simple phrase you're comfortable with 'I don't want to', or 'I'd rather not'.

- Calmly repeat your 'No' if the first one is not accepted. 'I hear what you're saying, but no, I'd rather not'.

Other tips

- Value yourself and value other people.

- Work out what you need and want out of life.

- Be prepared to compromise.

- Keep to any point you're making – don't let others distract you from it.

- Keep your voice slow, steady and low-pitched, and stay relaxed.

A problem shared

All of us need someone who cares about us and who is interested in what we do. This can bring comfort and relief and can even prevent us from feeling down or stressed in the first place. A problem shared really is a problem halved. However, be careful only to confide in those you can trust. This can be a member of your family, a friend, a colleague or one of the many support groups which are there waiting to help. It is not a sign of weakness to seek such support. It can be a massive help and it is a real strength to recognize this.

> *MYTH: Mothers with PND just need to pull themselves together and get on with it.*
>
> **FACT:** Mothers with PND are constantly trying to do this, but they simply can't. You might as well 'pull yourself together' to stop a heart attack, or cure a broken ankle.

I fell pregnant just after I split with my boyfriend. We'd only been together for six months. He doesn't even know about the baby. But I was pleased. I'd been really broody for a baby and my mum was a great support when I was pregnant and when the baby came. I thought I was doing really well but then the depression started – and the agitation. I just couldn't wind down and relax. Mum gave me this magazine and it had breathing exercises in it. She said I should try it. I thought how stupid can that be? To please mum, I tried it, and it actually helped me. Now I use it every day. Such a lovely feeling.

Sarah, 19

*I had PND with all three of my
children. I took antidepressants each
time and they really helped. But with
my last baby, I wanted to feel that I was
doing something too. Not just waiting
for the pills to work. My partner looked
after the children one night a week so
that I could go to a beginners' Salsa
class at the community centre. It was
such a laugh and I made some new
friends too. Just getting out for a while
with the music and the exercise seemed
to give me such a lift.*

Lee, 29

I've always been a bit of a free spirit. Very spontaneous. My partner is just the same. Having a baby was a bit like that. I had a sudden enthusiasm for being a mother. We were both so excited about this new experience, especially when little Joe was born. But of course it's hard to be a free spirit and do anything on the spur of the moment when you have a new baby. Don't get me wrong, we both love Joe more than I can say. But while I was adjusting to my new life, I felt so low and so trapped by the routine of it all. I'm glad to say that things are getting better now. We went on a weekend retreat a couple of months ago, with other parents dealing with similar issues, and that was a huge help.

Annie, 31

Summary of main self-help points

- Slow down and relax at some point every day.

- Make sure you are breathing in a relaxed way.

- Take breaks regularly.

- Cushion yourself with regular healthy meals or snacks, lots of sleep, enjoyable exercise and leisure.

- Take control of the panic attacks.

- Watch out for your thinking habits.

- Sort out your anger.

- Become more assertive if necessary.

- Share your troubles.

9

The recovery process
– first weeks
and beyond

In this final chapter of Part 2 we concentrate on what you can expect in terms of the postnatal depression (PND) recovery process. You are bound to have many questions and we'll try to answer them all for you. However, this is a really big subject, so if we miss anything that you want to know, remember you can contact any of the organizations or helplines given in Part 5, or ask your doctor or health visitor. In this chapter we will also give you some further help with keeping that important bond with your baby as strong as it can be.

How long will it be until you are yourself again?

It will reassure you to know that with appropriate treatment you can expect to make a full recovery. How long this takes will vary a lot from woman to woman, so it is difficult to give you a definite answer to this question. We are probably talking about months rather than weeks to return completely to your old self again. A lot will depend on how ill you are feeling to begin with and the treatment you go for. As we've said, it can often take a bit of trial and error before you settle for a particular antidepressant, and finding the best dosage for you can take a little time too. If you opt for 'talking treatment', there may be a waiting list, so this will inevitably take a bit longer.

Q. How will I know when I've fully recovered?

A. Good question. It's quite hard to put your finger on this. It can creep up on you when you're not looking for it. You usually know afterwards, but maybe not at the time. For example, you might suddenly realize that you haven't had any problems for a couple of weeks or a month or so. And that's it. It's gone.

What will happen if you don't have treatment?

As we've explained earlier in the book, even without treatment, PND usually gets better in time, although it may take up to a year or more. Although most women will recover completely and never experience depression again, some women who did not have their PND treated have found that the low feelings and anxiety can return a few years later, sometimes more than once. Untreated PND can also mean a lot of needless suffering for you and your family. It will spoil your experience of being a new mother and undermine the relationship with your baby and partner – not to mention how ill you can feel yourself. The sooner you are your old self again, the better. If you do decide on treatment, whatever you choose, this should considerably shorten your recovery time and make life bearable again. It should also reduce the chance of depression returning later.

Pattern of recovery – what to expect

Just as there is no set length to the recovery process, there is no set pattern for how it may feel for you going through it. There will be similarities with other women, but there will also be differences, so don't be alarmed if you talk to someone who has got better more quickly than you, or who describes a completely different set of experiences. You should receive more detail of what to expect from the therapist or from your doctor if you take medication. The leaflets provided with the medication can be particularly detailed and informative but, of course, never hesitate to ask if you are uncertain or want to know something. Making contact with other women in the various support groups, both locally and on the internet, can help to give a much broader picture of women's experiences. Part 4 of this book also gives you examples of other women's experiences in more depth.

The main thing to be aware of, which doesn't vary, is that your recovery will be very gradual. You can start to feel a little better within a week or two of starting any treatment, and then progress from there. You may have good days and bad days within this gradual improvement, so don't be put off by a bad day. You may even have ups and downs within the same day. Many women with depression feel at their worst first thing in the morning, but then improve slowly as the day progresses. You may also find you have occasional setbacks lasting a few days or even a week or more. Again, don't be put off by this, just keep going. These setbacks can and do happen, but they don't mean you are getting worse again or that you won't recover. We'll explain a lot more about setbacks in Part 3, Chapter 10, but just keep this at the back of your mind for now.

MYTH: Once you've had PND, you're never the same happy person again.

FACT: It does take a bit of time, but you can and will get back to your old self.

How long will you be on medication?

Like everything else about PND, this will vary. It could be for a year or more. It is certainly likely to take between eight and nine months until you feel really better. However, you shouldn't stop there. It is not uncommon to take antidepressants for at least six months after you start to feel really better. This may sound like a long time, but don't be in a hurry. If you come off the medication too soon, your PND may return. It's best to be on the safe side with this kind of thing. If you have had PND or depression before, you may need to be on medication for a bit longer.

Your brain chemistry has a very delicate balance and needs to be treated gently and with kid gloves. You should have regular visits to your doctor for check-ups, and he will advise you on when to change or cut down your medication. We'll explain a lot more about coming off your pills in Part 3, Chapter 10.

How long does 'talking treatment' take?

Putting the waiting time aside, this is likely to take some months to have its full effect and, like medication, will be a gradual process. There may be ten or more sessions to attend, with maybe two or three weeks in between, so this may well take a bit of time. You can probably expect to begin to feel better gradually after the first few sessions.

Q. How long does it take to get better?

A. You'll find that this varies a lot from person to person, depending on how ill you've been, how long you've had PND and how long it takes to get the right treatment for you. But it is likely to be months rather than weeks.

Keeping the bond with your baby strong during recovery

We've already touched on your concerns about bonding with your baby and have suggested that you have as much everyday contact with your baby as you can. The bond can develop through every one of her senses – through touch, eye contact, the sound of your voice and even the way you smell. So make sure to hold her close and talk to your baby whenever you can. Remember, it doesn't matter if you don't feel anything to start with, just go through the motions and a spark will eventually kindle.

It is important for you both that you can make that bond as strong as it can be. This will be good for the baby's development and also for your peace of mind. **You can fall in love with your baby at any time, not just in the first moments or days.** It's never too late to form that strong attachment and the feeling that you would do anything to protect her. As you begin to feel a little better, this will all become much easier.

To help that bond grow and strengthen, you could also try massaging your baby. This can help to bring the two of you closer and will also help you both to relax. It's a really good way to spend quality time with a small baby. This may sound a bit odd, but massaging babies, and their mothers too, has been a common practice in many parts of the world for hundreds of years.

How to massage your baby

Make sure that you have a bit of time available when you won't be disturbed and, most importantly, make sure that the room is warm. You can put on some relaxing music, too, if you like. You may find trying this out on a doll or a teddy helps you to get used to the idea and gain a little confidence. If you still feel anxious, try using one of the relaxation or breathing exercises we gave you in Chapter 3, before you start.

It's best not to do this if the baby seems unwell or has recently been immunized or had some other form of treatment.

Undress your baby, but leave a clean nappy under her, or to hand, for accidents. Check your hands are nicely warm. Maybe rub them together and shake them to loosen them up. Your baby will come to associate this with a massage coming. You can use a little baby oil on your hands if you find this makes it easier, but it helps to warm it a little if you decide to use it.

It's important not to use any other type of oil, such as aromatherapy oils. Keep talking to your baby while you're going through all these preparations, make eye contact and tell her that you're going to give her a lovely massage.

Now **gently** begin to stroke any part of your baby's body – except for your baby's tummy if she's under four weeks old. If you feel confident with it, and your baby is content with it, you can turn her over and do her back, but avoid massaging her spine. If your baby isn't enjoying any part of the massage, then stop what you're doing and move on. If she is enjoying something, you can stay with that a little longer.

Massage can help your baby to sleep better and can even relieve colic, so it has many advantages if you decide to try it out. If you want to learn more about it, ask your health visitor, or contact the National Childbirth Trust or International Association of Infant Massage (contact details in Part 5). There are local groups and local classes in many parts of the country.

Keeping everybody on side as you recover

At first, once you've explained things to them, everyone around you is likely to be very supportive and enthusiastic and be a huge help to you. However, like everything else, they can begin to forget and let things slip a bit, especially after a few weeks or months have gone by. It may be that you find yourself on your own a lot again, or doing all the housework and all the childcare again, with no 'me-time' or relaxation time. Friends may stop calling to ask how you're doing, or to ask you to join them on outings. It won't be deliberate, and can easily happen, especially if you are beginning to sound and feel more like your old self again. Try not to be angry or resentful about this but remember that it wouldn't be happening if you weren't feeling and sounding a little better.

It helps to keep everybody on side if you can be ready to ask for the help you need – but in a warm and understanding way. Don't be tempted to slip into nagging everyone around you and 'playing the PND card'. You are all in this together. See it as a team effort and just give them a gentle but encouraging reminder like, 'Taking me out to the shops last week was a huge help. I really appreciated it. When can we do it again?' Let them know that their help has made a huge impact on your recovery so far and let them know how much you value and appreciate their help and support.

Keep PND on the agenda all the time, without being a nag or a bore. Give them updates on how you're feeling but don't wait to be asked. **You** make the phone call or text the friends who haven't been in touch for a while. People are busy and they do have many other commitments, so keep in touch, but keep it up-beat and stay positive. If you are having a bad day or a setback, it will be obvious to them, and you won't have to remind them that you still need them.

MYTH: If I tell my friends how I'm feeling about my baby, they'll never speak to me again.

FACT: You will be surprised at how many of your friends will know and understand more about PND than you think. PND is nothing to be ashamed of. And, after all, what are friends for?

How other mothers with PND can help

When family and friends are beginning to forget a little, and run out of enthusiasm, you will find that other mothers with PND can be a constant and reliable source of support. They won't forget about you and they won't stop offering help and being there for you as a listening and supportive ear. They will continue to understand when others just can't, or haven't the time or energy.

So, from the start, it helps if you can have regular contact with other mums you know, or with a support group in your area. If this isn't possible or available, there is lots of support on the internet or telephone. As we've said, having PND is something you can't really understand if you haven't been there. It can be such a relief and an enormous support to share your feelings with someone who really knows what you're talking about. Any woman who has had depression at any time in her life will be able to understand. That's why we can understand. We have both had depression ourselves.

I had PND after my twins were born. I already had a little girl of three, and it was so hard to cope. I didn't go to the doctor until it got really bad. I had it after the first birth, but it was quite mild, and it passed after about two months without me doing anything. This time was really different. Telling my mother and sister was awful, but I really needed their help. I'd broken up with my partner and was living on my own, but they were great, really stood by me. They helped out with shopping and the babies, and all sorts. They both help whenever they can now, and I know that all I need to do is ask.

Lisa, 38

I had really bad PND when my son, Jason, was born. I'm a lone parent, and Jason's dad just doesn't want to know. I was lucky though as the health visitor spotted it really quickly. She also showed me how to massage Jason. I felt really stupid at first, but she said it would help me and Jason. I had been feeling really distant from Jason and it really helped me to chill out. I had been so tense all the time and I got this lovely close feeling for the first time. It was great.

Yolanda, 19

Moving on to Part 3

We have now covered a lot of ground together and we appreciate how difficult it can be to concentrate. It's now time to finish off this part and move on to Part 3, where we'll tell you what to expect in the longer term. We'll also address any concerns you may have about this happening again with another pregnancy and any worries you may have about why this has happened to you, but not to many of your friends. Was there anything you could have done to prevent it? Did anything make you more vulnerable to PND? We'll also describe some of the complications and more serious conditions associated with childbirth.

Part 3:
Long-term
Challenges and
Future Hopes

10

Picking up the pieces
and getting back
to normal

What you will want more than anything is for life to get back to normal again. This third part of the book brings together a number of topics which will be relevant to you later on in your journey to recovery. In this chapter we tell you more about the process of coming off your pills and we give you some ideas on how to cope with the inevitable low moments and bad days along the way. We also address any concerns you may still have if the intimate side of your life is not yet back to normal. In Chapter 11 we get to grips with your worries about why postnatal depression (PND) has happened to you, and any fears you may have about it happening again. Chapter 12 covers some other possible psychological conditions which can occasionally develop from PND or which can accompany having a baby. To finish off this part, Chapter 13 takes a look back at the journey so far, and provides you with more reassurance, hints and tips to give you added strength and energy, to keep you going on your way back to full health.

The road to recovery

As soon as you start to deal with your PND, whether by talking therapy or pills, you should begin to move slowly but surely along that road to recovery. As we've explained already, you can expect this to be a gradual process over a number of months, with ups and downs along the way. It can take a huge effort to keep going along this road, especially when you have been so very tired, so you can be justly proud of what you have managed to achieve so far. When you are depressed it is much easier to take the line of least resistance, and do nothing at all. Making an effort, and doing anything else, can seem like a huge mountain to climb every day – and when you are depressed, that's just what it is.

Over those weeks and months since the baby was born, you will have found strength you didn't know you had to deal with this unexpected enemy, your PND. Recognize this, and give yourself a pat on the back, and maybe even a reward every so often. Buy those earrings you like or get your nails done, or have a night out. You deserve it. Of course, just feeling better can be a huge reward in itself, and as each week passes, you will begin to feel more and more like your old self.

> **MYTH:** *If I start taking antidepressants, I'll never get off them.*
>
> **FACT:** Most women find they have no problems coming off antidepressants, provided it is done very gradually and at the right time.

At first, you may get occasional flashes of feeling 'normal' again, only for a few seconds, or a few minutes out of the blue. And how wonderful those snatched moments will feel. You had forgotten what feeling normal felt like, just having that everyday contentment and feeling that things are all right with the world. To begin with, these snatched moments may be short and disappear just as mysteriously as they came. Then they will begin to happen more often, and then maybe last for a whole morning or for an afternoon. Then you might even find yourself looking forward to something, and that may be something you haven't done in a very long time.

If you had been struggling to bond with your baby, there will be a similar gradual improvement, with your relationship growing stronger day by day and meaning more and more to you both. You may have begun by going through the motions, as we suggested earlier in the book, but little by little, you will have begun to feel something, and those feelings will have strengthened and will give you such pleasure and reassurance. Your baby will have responded to this, too, by interacting with you more. Sometimes the bond can form suddenly, knocking you for six one day when he smiles at you or grabs your hair with his little fingers, or stops crying just because you picked him up. Just like that, you've bonded, and love has arrived at last. How good that feels.

Q. What is an episiotomy?

A. An episiotomy is an incision, or cut made between the vagina and the back passage to increase the opening of the vagina to prevent tearing and make the delivery of the baby easier. It will usually need to be stitched after the birth.

Coping with setbacks

It would be wrong of us to paint a completely rosy picture of constant improvement and progress when you are recovering from PND. Just like with many things in life, you are likely to experience ups and downs right from the start, and all the way through. You may already have experienced this. Some women are lucky and everything goes really smoothly, and it may be that you are one of the lucky ones. However, many women find the journey can be a bumpy one and you can find your mood changes over a day. This is quite common, as depression often has a daily pattern of being much worse in the morning, and then improving as the day goes on, though a few people do find the night-time is the worst.

Recovering from a condition which affects your mood is going to be like that, and it is much better to be prepared for these things. One day everything just slots into place, while on other days you can't seem to do anything right, and all the effort you're making seems like a waste of time. The encouraging news is that the bad day soon passes, to be replaced by a number of better more hopeful and more useful days, when you'll take another step forward and have a more positive attitude to life.

So don't be put off by the occasional bad day or even a more lengthy setback. These are all part and parcel of this illness. They are not your fault, setbacks can happen if you're physically unwell or run down. After a bout of the flu or another virus you should take extra care of yourself, as you will be especially vulnerable to a setback. You can overdo things and expect too much of yourself as you begin to feel a little better. Maybe there are new stresses in your life. Even after weeks and months of feeling better, your life stressors can increase out of the blue, sometimes without you noticing it, and you can feel anxious and down again. You can even just have an off day or two for no apparent reason.

Q. What is ovulation?

A. Ovulation is the release of a single, tiny egg from one of your ovaries. Once released, the egg is capable of being fertilized for 12 to 24 hours. If the released egg is fertilized and successfully implants in your womb, it results in pregnancy. If the egg is not fertilized, it is passed out during menstrual bleeding, which starts about two weeks after ovulation.

The key thing is to be vigilant, and always on the look out for signs that things are not improving quite as they should be. If this does happen to you, just make sure that you stay on track, keep taking your medication or following your talking treatment programme, and soon all will feel better again. Stick with it, and we promise that you'll soon be back on top of things again. Coping with setbacks is all part of the recovery process.

Q. I had PND with my first baby. Is there an ideal time to wait before having another baby?

A. There has been no research undertaken in this area, but it would probably be best to wait until you are feeling completely well again, and aim for a time when you are well prepared for another baby and there is minimum stress in your life.

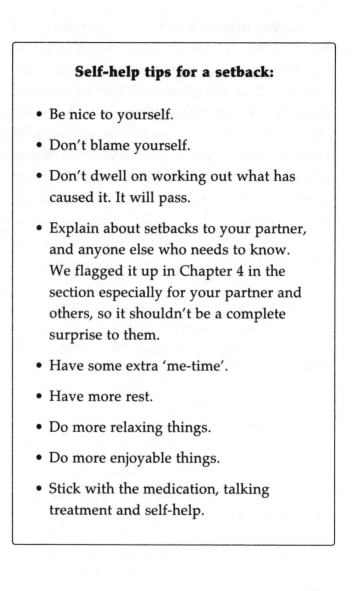

Self-help tips for a setback:

- Be nice to yourself.

- Don't blame yourself.

- Don't dwell on working out what has caused it. It will pass.

- Explain about setbacks to your partner, and anyone else who needs to know. We flagged it up in Chapter 4 in the section especially for your partner and others, so it shouldn't be a complete surprise to them.

- Have some extra 'me-time'.

- Have more rest.

- Do more relaxing things.

- Do more enjoyable things.

- Stick with the medication, talking treatment and self-help.

Your sex life to be

A common effect of depression is a complete loss of interest in sex. This may last for some time, and it will help if both you and your partner realize that this is a symptom of the illness, and that sexual desire and your libido will return gradually as you recover. Having as much physical contact as you can, like simple touching, hugging and cuddling, can do much to reassure you both and prepare the way for full sexual desire to return. It helps to remember that your

---

MYTH: You can't get pregnant when you are breastfeeding.

FACT: You can get pregnant when you are breastfeeding. There can be many months when you can't because you are not ovulating, but when you begin to ovulate again, you will be fertile again before you have your first period.

Q. What does 'libido' mean?

A. Libido is another word for your sexual drive or sexual appetite. It varies from one person to another. Your libido can also change over time, and is strongly influenced by your circumstances at the time.

partner is likely to be missing your usual intimacy very much, and this may be proving very difficult for him to cope with.

It can take some months to resume your normal sex life with your partner. It's not just you this can happen to. Every new mother will need time to adjust back to having sex again and being able to really enjoy it. It's not only the obvious physical reasons that mean that this takes a bit of time, it can take a long time after a birth for you to feel like sex, or feel sexy again. You now have very different associations with your vagina and your breasts, and this can have quite an inhibiting effect on many women, and incidentally on some men too. It can take you both some time to readjust, but it will happen.

You will also be much more tired than before and, with a new baby, and perhaps other children in the house, finding times in your day when you and your partner can really relax and enjoy each other's bodies can become more difficult. Spontaneity can disappear completely, as you find you have to take advantage of the moment when it appears, rather than being able to make love whenever and wherever you want. If that spontaneity and variety was part of the excitement for you, it can be difficult to get that same spark when you have to be more deliberate and cold-heartedly sensible about when and where you have sex. You may have had time for lots of build-up and foreplay and both really enjoyed and needed that part of love-making in order for you to orgasm. However, with a baby around, you may only have a few rushed minutes available, and you may not really be in the mood. It can feel like pressure and all this contributes to a much less satisfactory sex life for many parents.

You may well still be struggling with all this, even a year or more after the birth, and this only adds to any loss of libido you are having due to your PND. Bear in mind that many antidepressants can reduce your libido, too, or make orgasm more difficult to achieve. So check out the list of side effects with your pills and, if you are badly affected by this, you might be able to change to another pill which suits you better. Also, don't forget to think about contraception when you start having sex again. It is possible to get pregnant before your periods return.

In the meantime, here are some suggestions which may help to increase desire and increase opportunities:

Tips to re-awaken sexual feelings

- Plan a time when you can be sure to get together to make love. Your mother or a friend might take the baby and the other children overnight, or for an afternoon.

- Do make sure you've talked about it, and neither of you feels under pressure to make love. You can still have a great time without actually having sex.

- Try to get into the mood. Make it special. Soft music, candles, a relaxed meal and a glass of wine can all help to re-awaken that side of you both.

- Start gradually with the pleasures of everyday stroking and touching, before you move on to sexual touching, or take time out before you make love to relax in the bath and pamper yourself or share a massage first.

- Make time to talk to each other. Your relationship needs to be pampered regularly to encourage sexual feelings.

Coming off the pills

We've discussed a bit about this in Chapter 7, but it is later on in the recovery process when you will really need to know about coming off your pills. Here are some main points to remember. We apologize if we are repeating anything we said earlier, but these points are all so important:

- Stick with your medication, even on the bad days. Bad days don't mean the medication isn't working.

- Take your pills every day – if you miss even one day, you can get symptoms recurring, but don't take twice your normal medication in any one day to compensate.

- Ask your doctor or health visitor for advice about when and how to come off your medication. Don't go it alone.

- Don't come off your pills as soon as you are feeling a little better. You have to wait until you feel **completely** back to your self again – **and then wait another few months**.

- When you do start to come off your pills, you must do this very gradually. Gradually means really slowly, cutting down over a number of months. For example, you might reduce from four pills a day to three for about a month, then if all is well, go down to two for another month, and so on. Each medication will be slightly different so ask for advice.

- If you find your symptoms coming back, tell the doctor straight away. You may be trying to come off too early.

- A few women find that they can come off the pills successfully and feel fine for a number of months, but then they can begin to feel depressed again, and have to have a few more months on the medication again. This is all just part and parcel of the illness, so be patient.

Q. Are you more likely to have PND with a boy or a girl?

A. There is no evidence to suggest that the sex of your baby makes any difference to the likelihood of you having PND.

Withdrawal symptoms when coming off pills

Just as it took a week or two for your body to adjust when you started taking your pills, you are likely to feel the effects of cutting down your medication, even if you do this gradually. So don't be put off if you feel a little off colour when you reduce your dosage. You might have a bit of a stomach upset, flu like symptoms, or dizziness. You might also have more frequent and very vivid dreams, and the occasional strange feeling for a while. Read the leaflet which comes with your pills before you start to reduce the dosage, so that you know what to expect. Not everyone has these effects, and they should wear off after a few days, so stick with it. You'll get there.

Sometimes, the effects of withdrawing can be similar to the original problem. You might feel a bit tense, anxious or down. If this happens don't worry unduly. This is quite common and will usually pass after a day or two. If things don't improve, or you have any other signs of your PND returning, speak to the doctor straight away as you may be trying to come off too early. It can sometimes take a little time to get all of this right, so don't be discouraged. You will get there.

Depression can happen at any time

Something else we should alert you to is that depression can happen at any time. It doesn't only happen when you have had a baby. There are many occasions in life when stress can make you feel anxious and down. Sometimes you can become depressed completely out of the blue, and you won't be able to pin down a cause. If you've had PND, there is a small chance that you may become depressed again. This is discouraging, we know, but it won't necessarily happen to you. It just pays to be on the alert, so that it can be nipped in the bud. If you feel any of those old familiar symptoms, go straight to the doctor for help. The sooner it is dealt with the sooner you will recover again. This is where your partner, family and friends can continue to help, too, so keep them on side, and encourage them to let you know if they notice any signs of depression returning. They can sometimes spot these things before you can. There is more on this in Chapter 12.

Getting back to normal

As things begin to improve, don't forget to start to pick up the pieces of your life. There will be friends you haven't seen for a long time and who will be wondering what has happened to you. Some of them may not even have seen the new baby. There will be special occasions you've had to miss because you weren't feeling up to it, and you'll have old leisure pursuits and interests which were abruptly dropped. Don't try to do everything at once, but do start picking up on things where you left off. Give people a call and explain you're feeling better and can have a coffee or a drink sometime. Maybe have a meal together. Explain about your PND if you feel you want to, but you don't have to. You can say that you've not been too well, or that the baby has taken up a lot of your time. Write those overdue thank you letters for baby gifts. It's never too late for these. You'll have all the time in the world, so no need to rush it. Just do one or two things every week. That will be enough.

The midwife gave me a leaflet about PND when my son was born four years ago, so I was on the look out for it happening to me. But it didn't and I had a wonderful experience. Then when Sam was three, I started to get really irritable and moody, and just lost interest in everything. The house was a mess and I couldn't be bothered with anything. I blamed myself and thought I was a lazy, useless human being. I would still be thinking that now if it hadn't been for my smear test visit to the nurse. She just asked me how I was, and I broke down and sobbed. I didn't know that you could have depression any time, not just after you have a baby.

Nina, 23

Having PND was the worst experience of my life. Impossible to put it into words. I can't describe the relief when I began to feel better week by week. So, it was such a terrible shock when I had a setback. It came completely from nowhere. I just woke up one morning and all the symptoms were back. Everything. I cried and cried and cried. My mother phoned the doctor and the health visitor came round later that day. It was such a relief to find out that this can happen, and it didn't mean I wasn't going to get better. I can't even begin to describe how I felt that day. Thankfully, within a few days, I was myself again.

Rani, 28

11

What about another pregnancy?

When you are beginning to feel more like your old self again, or maybe before that, you'll begin to wonder about what might happen if you have another baby. Having postnatal depression (PND) is the kind of experience you don't want to repeat. So you will be wondering about your next pregnancy. You may be asking 'Why did this happen to me?' You may even be thinking that you won't have any more children. In this chapter we will try to answer your questions about what might happen with another pregnancy, and maybe even give you some idea of why you have had PND this time around. We'll also tell you about the preventative treatments that are available and suggest how you might best prepare for another pregnancy.

Could you have done anything to stop yourself getting PND?

Hindsight is a wonderful thing, and we have no doubt that after reading this book, you will think of things you could have done to make it less likely you would have PND. But you didn't have the benefit of hindsight then. You didn't know. Making a difference next time has to do with many things, and we will explain these in this chapter. You must remember though, that there are no guarantees. If nothing you do makes any difference, and you are still unlucky enough to have PND next time, at least you will know what to look out for, and you will recognize it straight away if it happens. You will also know what to do to get help and get better. Catching these things early can make all the difference in the world.

> *MYTH: If you have PND with one baby you will have it with every baby.*
>
> **FACT:** You are a bit more likely to have PND again if you've had it once, but it is by no means certain. Many women only have it once.

Should you do anything differently with your next pregnancy?

If you have PND with one baby, you may well be more likely to have PND with your next baby. We don't really know how high the risk is though, because there are no accurate statistics on how likely this is. It is probably best to be prepared in case you become ill after your next birth. You can do this by making sure that you will have plenty of support immediately after the baby is born, and that you have organized some help with caring for your older children. If you have it in mind that you may become ill, you will be able to get treatment quickly should you notice depression symptoms. Early detection and early treatment are both factors, which previous sufferers have in their favour. On the other hand, things may go completely normally, and you may sail through this birth and the months after it. Many women do.

If you do have PND again

If you do have PND again, and we really hope that you don't, then at least you will recognize it whenever it appears this time. First time around, it can take a long time to realize that something is actually wrong, and an even longer time to do something about it. Early mild signs may not even be noticed first time, but will be important warning signs to look out for again, and should sound the alarm. So you will get help much, much sooner, and that can make such a huge difference, not just to you, but to your partner, your baby and your whole family. You'll also know which is the best medication for you, or whether talking treatment was more suited to you. If you had talking treatment the first time, this may even prepare you for coping if the condition occurs again. Your partner, family and friends will be much easier to recruit to help you, as they already know the ropes. Although it won't be a bed of roses, it should at least be less of a trauma than it was the first time and, with luck, it should clear up much faster, letting you get back to your old self again sooner.

Does anything make PND more likely?

Anyone, but anyone can have PND. You will almost certainly know someone who has had it, and you will also have heard many celebrities talking about having it. These include Katie Price (model, also known as Jordan), Suzanne Shaw (from 'Hear Say'), Fern Britton (TV Presenter), Natasha Hamilton (from 'Atomic Kitten'), Gail Porter (TV presenter) and Denise Welch (actress). Some of these celebrities will be giving you a 'message of hope' in Part 4.

Some people are undoubtedly more vulnerable than others to developing PND. This is down to many different factors and circumstances.

MYTH: There's nothing you can do to prevent having PND.

FACT: There is lots you can do if you think you may be at risk. There are self-help strategies as well as medical and psychological preventative treatments.

According to the charity MAMA, research has shown that there are a number of factors which may make some women more vulnerable to developing PND. These factors include:

- A family history of depression or PND.

- Previously having had PND.

- Depression during the pregnancy.

- Having no one to confide in.

- Having a poor relationship with your own mother or partner.

- Major life events in the 12 months before the birth (for example, bereavement, moving house, or unemployment).

- The pregnancy being unplanned.

- Financial, or other worries.

- A traumatic birth experience.

- Being physically unwell after the birth.

Don't beat yourself up about how many of these factors may have applied to you with this baby, and so probably played a part in your developing PND. You weren't to know. Why should you have known? **You were in no way responsible.** Most of these factors are completely out of your control, but having read this book you will be much better prepared for another baby when the time comes.

There is no need to panic too much at this list and what it might mean for another baby. Many of us could tick any number of these factors. Remember these factors only **increase the risk**. None of them means that you will definitely have PND. Some may only slightly increase the risk. This is by no means an exact science. Having had PND before, or having depression in the family, does not mean that it is definitely going to happen to you with a first baby, or that it will happen again with a second or subsequent birth.

That said, these are factors to be aware of, and you should minimize their effects if you can. You can't change your previous experiences, or your family background, but there are many factors that you can work on changing or reducing their effects in your next pregnancy. Much of this is covered in the 'self-help' preparing for pregnancy section later in this chapter.

Treatment to prevent PND

As we mentioned earlier, in Chapter 7, if you have a history of PND, your doctor may prescribe the hormone progesterone as a way of preventing it recurring. This is given by injection immediately after birth, and then in gradually smaller amounts over the next week or so. You then need to use progesterone pessaries until your periods start again. This treatment is relatively new, and may not be available everywhere, so ask your doctor if you want to know more. It should be stressed that this treatment is as yet unproven but early results indicate that it can be helpful in some cases. There is also some evidence that extra 'psychological' support during a subsequent pregnancy reduces the likelihood of an episode of PND. Your doctor or health visitor may be able to arrange this for you.

The other method involves the use of antidepressants in late pregnancy, usually in the last three weeks. Some doctors feel that exposing the baby to antidepressants even in late pregnancy is dangerous. However, others feel that the benefit to the mother outweighs the risk to the baby. This is something to spend time thinking about, and to discuss at length with your doctor.

Preparing for another pregnancy

Here are some helpful suggestions to help you prepare for another pregnancy, and the kinds of things you can do for yourself to reduce the chance of having PND. It is important to realize that these are in no way being suggested as an alternative to medical treatment. These are just common sense precautions, which are worth taking.

There are of course no guarantees. We are in the realm of risks and probabilities, not certainties. We know that this is difficult for you, but until there is more research done, and more definite information around, this is the best we can do. This is a good reason for keeping in contact with a support group, as they will be aware of any new preventative treatments, and also be able to advise on how effective these might be.

Probably the first and most important thing to do before trying for another baby is to have a long chat with your doctor or health visitor or, if you prefer, a local self-help group or one of the helplines given in Part 5. They will give you the up-to-date thinking on preparing for a pregnancy and will also be able to give advice and information which is tailored to you in particular, with your history, and your circumstances. No two women are going to be exactly the same. If you need some counselling to come to a decision about whether to proceed with another pregnancy, your doctor may be able to arrange this for you.

Do allow plenty of time for this kind of detective work to take place before you even start to try for a baby. You may have to wait a bit longer, too, to get the circumstances just right. You may be moving house, for example, and it's better to avoid that kind of stress around this time. So try to be clear of major stresses for at least 12 months before you become pregnant, and for at least a year after. Impossible, you may think – you can't control what happens in your life. We understand that but, in so far as you can, avoid such stresses you have direct control over, such as moving house, having a new kitchen fitted, taking on a new job or promotion, or getting married. Choose to do these things some other time. They can wait. Having your baby and enjoying every moment of the experience is much more important for now.

If you are reading this book before you have your first baby, because you feel at risk, or because you just want to know more about PND, you could also use any of the ideas given here.

You could also think about spending time with a new mum and see what it's really like. Don't just meet for a coffee, but spend a whole day or a weekend with her to find out what it can be like all day every day, and possibly with a broken night too. Do lots of babysitting, and not just in the evening when the baby is asleep, to get a taste of what being alone for hours with a baby can be like. That way you'll experience both the joys and the hard work and restrictions that being a mother can bring, and you'll be so much better prepared when your own baby arrives.

Whether this is first time around for you or not, having lots of support around you is really important. Make sure you have someone you can share your feelings with. Your partner, a good friend, your mother or an aunt, maybe a sister. If there is no one obvious around, maybe join a mothers' group before the baby arrives, such as the UK's National Childbirth Trust (NCT), for example, or any other sort of women's group. If there is a Women's centre in your area go along and see what's available there. Support like this can act as a kind of protection or cushion against anxiety and depression.

Do make certain that you will have help around the house just after the birth when you are tired and adjusting to the changes in your life. You may feel that you can cope with all of that second time around – you've already been there and done that – but having a second baby is never the same as having your first. No two babies are ever the same, and having two children is not just double the work and disruption of one, the upheaval and workload is usually much more than the sum of the parts, and can still come as quite a surprise.

Try to adopt as healthy a lifestyle as possible all the way from trying for the baby, through the pregnancy and after the birth, as this will give you terrific protection against ill health of all kinds, including stress and PND. So keep fit and active, make sure you are well rested with lots of good quality sleep, find time for regular breaks and some fun, and eat a healthy well-balanced diet, preferably with at least three meals a day. All easy to say, but you will need enthusiasm and commitment to have a lifestyle like this. The effort will all be worthwhile.

If you can, avoid an unplanned pregnancy, as this can cause major stress, making you much more vulnerable to ill health of all kinds. It also has knock-on effects on other factors which may make PND more likely. You won't have had any choice in the timing, for example, so it may all come at a very awkward time. Your relationship with your partner will possibly suffer if he wasn't thinking of another baby at that time, or you may be without a partner if the baby is the outcome of a short relationship. Keep an eye on your contraception regime, whatever it is, and don't let it slip when you are busy with your first baby. If your periods have not returned after the baby is born or because you are breastfeeding, don't rely on that for contraception. You can have ovulated and be fertile again before your first period arrives.

After the new baby is born, follow all the advice we have already given in Chapters 3 and 8, even if you are feeling well and happy. PND can develop months after a birth, so you have to look after yourself in the long term. You also need to look after yourself even after the risk of PND is over as you can feel stressed or have depression at any time, not just after a baby. Make our suggestions part of your way of life. Make sure you have time just for you, time just for your partner, keep active, stay positive and make time to relax. Not only will you enjoy life more, but you will be cushioned from the stresses and strains of life.

After my son was born six years ago, I had PND really badly. When I began to feel a bit better, I joined a local women's group. They had a health visitor come along to give a talk about how to prepare for pregnancy and reduce the chances of having PND. There were no guarantees, but I gave it a go with my second pregnancy. I followed the self-help suggestions she gave us while I was pregnant, and afterwards too. Maybe it was just luck, but my daughter is now nine months old, and so far so good.

Jamila, 30

We had just moved to a bigger house and taken on a bigger mortgage when I became pregnant for the first time. I lost my mother the year before and I missed having her around so much. After Josh was born, I was absolutely fine for about three months, and then one day I had an enormous panic attack. My husband is a doctor, so he knew straight away what the problem was, and I had 'talking therapy' straight away. It took a bit of time, but I did gradually recover. We both wanted at least one other child, but I was really scared. What if it happened again? During the 'talking treatment' we had talked about all the stress that had been in my life just before I got pregnant with Josh, and how maybe that had played a part in me having PND. Things were quite relaxed at that time, no major stresses in our lives, so we tried for a baby again, and I couldn't believe it, everything was okay this time. No sign at all of PND.

Sonia, 33

12

Other conditions that can occasionally develop

In this chapter we hope to raise your awareness of some of the other possible conditions that can develop after you've had a baby, but we don't want you to start worrying about these. These are all relatively unusual, some very rare and unlikely. We just want you to be alert to any signs of these, so that you can get treatment quickly, should they appear. Early help will considerably shorten these conditions, and we can assure you now that all of them are treatable.

Recurrent bouts of depression

Some women who have had PND have found that bouts of depression can return later on, months or years later, sometimes more than once. You know already how long it can take for a bout like this to lift, so you can find yourself feeling out of sorts for many weeks, with all the difficulties that can bring. This can be so discouraging and it's not easy for partners, family or friends either.

It may be that this is more likely to happen if you don't have treatment for your PND when you first experience it. Many women have found this. It is probable that having your PND treated now will make this much less likely to happen. It's also a good idea to keep up the self-help lifestyle after you are fully recovered from your PND. It is, after all, just a healthy lifestyle, so it will have lots of other benefits for you and the family too. If it can also help to prevent you becoming depressed again, that is a huge extra bonus.

What this also means is that it will still be important to keep your eyes open for any signs of the depression recurring some months or even years after you have recovered from PND. In the same way as it is important to spot the signs of PND and get treatment as soon as you can, the more quickly you are treated for this later bout of depression the better. There is no need to worry all the time about this. Just have it at the back of your mind. If you have treatment for your PND, it is unlikely that you will have any recurrences like this.

PND can sometimes lead to other conditions

There are some other conditions which a minority of mothers can develop through having PND, especially if their PND has not been diagnosed and treated. As you know, many mothers with PND will experience anxiety and panic attacks. In most women that's as far as it will go, and this will gradually disappear as they recover. However, for a few women, this can become a bit of a problem, and the panic attacks can persist even after the PND has lifted. Some women will even find that they begin to avoid situations in which they are afraid they might feel anxious or panicky. It's easy to understand how this can happen.

It may be that you find yourself making excuses for not going out with friends, or asking other people to get the shopping, because you don't like the way you feel in these situations. This won't cause a problem if it only happens occasionally and sorts itself out. It's only when this avoidance continues, and maybe becomes more frequent, that some women can go on to develop what is known as 'panic disorder' or 'anxiety disorder', depending on the kinds of situations which are being avoided.

Like PND, these are psychological or behavioural conditions and they are all treatable. If you do recognize any of these conditions, or are simply worried about any of them, now or in the future, do speak to your doctor straight away. As we've said, they are all treatable, and they will be sorted out more quickly if they are caught early on.

MYTH: People with a phobia are weak, cowardly people.

FACT: This can happen to absolutely anybody. It is not a sign of weakness or of being cowardly, in any way.

Phobias

As we've been explaining, having panic attacks can lead some women to begin to avoid situations in which they fear they may panic. A kind of 'fear of fear', as it is often called. Avoidance like this can easily lead to you developing a 'phobia'. Phobias are more common than you might think but, like PND, it's not something people tend to talk about. The phobias most likely to develop from PND are probably agoraphobia and social phobia. You may have heard these called 'irrational fear'. They are not at all irrational of course. What is at the bottom of it is the fear of suffering a panic attack or other unpleasant anxiety symptoms in public, or somewhere you can't easily leave, such as the theatre or school parents' evening. This is not an unreasonable, nor indeed an irrational, fear.

People are not actually afraid of going outside, or socializing with their friends; they fear these unpleasant anxiety symptoms, or being embarrassed in public when they have them. For the sufferer there is no logical explanation for the panic attack, so the attacks quickly become associated with where they happen, leading to a build-up of avoidance, and further anxiety.

The unconscious conclusion is that if no other explanation for the panic attack is forthcoming, it must have been something to do with where they were and what they were doing at the time. Sufferers can often feel that they must be going mad, but they aren't, of course. It's not only having PND which can bring on a phobia like this, people can develop a phobia for all sorts of reasons. The common factor would seem to be having anxiety or panicky feelings.

Social phobia

Social phobia can develop in a similar way to agoraphobia. The main difference is probably that the situation avoided is that of having to 'perform' in some way in front of one or more people. Having to have a conversation, dance, sign a document, give a talk or demonstration, or eat or drink may all become sources of embarrassment or fear if you have visible symptoms of anxiety such as blushing, shaking, sweating or panicking.

Agoraphobia

Q. What is agoraphobia?

A. Agoraphobia is often thought to be a fear of open spaces. This is not what agoraphobia is. It is literally 'fear of the market place'. It is a fear of crowded places and being away from home. You feel nervy, uncomfortable or panicky when you are out driving, walking or shopping or on public transport.

Often wrongly taken to be a fear of open spaces, agoraphobia is actually a fear of leaving the security of the home, particularly if you need to go to crowded places, wait in a queue or be in a group or audience of some kind. It is the symptoms experienced when outside which are feared, not being outside, in itself. Unpleasant symptoms experienced when out of the home become associated with being away from home, and a pattern of avoidance can develop.

Obsessive or compulsive behaviour

There are numerous harmless obsessions and compulsions and we all have them to some extent. Many people simply have to put a pinch of salt over their shoulder after spilling it, will not walk on the lines of the pavement or under a ladder, must have ornaments or books displayed in a certain way, or find themselves checking twice that the gas is off or the door is locked, even though they know they've just checked it. This is not a problem and is very common. However, when you are feeling tense and anxious, it's relatively easy to build up these habits and perhaps repeat things a little too often, or you can slip into unusual habits, which can reduce your anxiety and make you feel better, even temporarily. You might develop checking rituals, or little phrases you have to say at certain times, or find you wash your hands or tidy the house too thoroughly and too often.

This is normal behaviour taken just a bit too far. 'Compulsions' are behaviours which you can find yourself repeating to reduce anxiety. Whereas 'obsessions' usually refer to unwanted thoughts, ideas or impulses, which repeatedly recur in your mind.

Q. I'm always washing my hands now that the baby is here – after changes, before feeds, after putting out the rubbish. I've heard that might be OCD. What is OCD, and do I have it?

A. OCD is short for 'Obsessive Compulsive Disorder', and you are most unlikely to have it. As long as you feel that you are washing your hands in the usual way, and no more often than seems usual, you are absolutely fine. You do have to be careful with cleanliness when a baby is around. With OCD, people are repeatedly washing, cleaning, checking or carrying out some other habit, much more than they really know they should, and it will be interfering with their lives. For some people, they have thoughts which repeat in their heads much more than they should and also interfere with their lives.

Treatment for conditions

Even if you do develop one of these conditions, be assured that there is help available, and you will be able to cope again. There is much that can be done if you recognize yourself in any of the descriptions given so far in this chapter. Your doctor should be your first step. Recurrent panic attacks can often be treated with medication alone or with the help of a specially trained practice nurse or health visitor. Some practices have computer programmes you can follow and, in some areas, you may be offered 'bibliotherapy' which involves reading specially written and 'user-friendly' books, a bit like this one.

If you have begun to avoid situations, you may be offered help from a trained nurse or a psychologist, who will most often use techniques such as 'progressive desensitization' to treat you. This treatment is very similar to the 'talking treatment' we told you about in Chapter 7, but takes things further, helping you to very gradually relearn normal behaviour and thinking patterns.

For phobias, this involves a process of approaching the feared situation one step at a time, usually over several months. It would be very unusual for you to be forced to face your fears straight away, all at once. The agoraphobic person might begin by simply standing in the doorway and, once that is mastered through frequent practice, they will then progress to the end of the path, and so on. For obsessions and compulsions, you would be helped to gradually cut down on the compulsive piece of behaviour. In either case, relaxation and breathing exercises are used to reduce the feelings of anxiety produced by these small steps. Medication can also make a huge difference in most cases.

Should you experience any of these conditions, effective treatment is available for you. You don't need to feel embarrassed, and you shouldn't have to suffer in silence. Your doctor or your health visitor will completely understand and will be able to help you. There are also many support groups who can provide you with companionship, encouragement and information, and you'll find details of these in Part 5.

Postnatal Psychosis

For a very few women, there is a mental illness called Postnatal Psychosis (also called Puerperal Psychosis or Post-partum Psychosis) which can occur after having a baby. This serious illness needs urgent support and treatment. It is different from PND and affects around one in every 1,000 women, usually within days or weeks of childbirth. It causes rapid mood swings, strange or bizarre beliefs or hearing voices, and sufferers can behave in odd and unpredictable ways. Sufferers are unlikely to be aware they are behaving unusually or that they are ill, so they need immediate medical help and support. This may have to be in hospital, but it is usually possible for your baby to be with you while you recover. This illness is more likely to happen:

- If you have a family history of postnatal psychosis.

- If you have a family history of bipolar (manic-depressive) disorder.

- If you have bipolar disorder.

- If you had postnatal psychosis with a previous birth.

It is therefore important to let your doctor and midwife know about any of these factors while you are pregnant because they can adapt your treatment to reduce the risk of it happening. Although it is a serious condition, rest assured that with the proper treatment you can make a full recovery.

Q. I have a friend who is 'bipolar'. This used to be called manic depression. Is this the same as postnatal depression?

A. No. There are many forms of depression, but PND is quite different from manic depression, or 'bipolar disorder'. Bipolar disorder can happen any time, not just after a baby, and those that suffer from it have episodes where they feel really 'up' or 'high' for a few days or weeks and also suffer from periods of feeling really down and depressed.

Looking back on it now, it's all a bit unreal. I had these awful panic attacks. They tended to happen whenever I was in the supermarket, especially at the check-out. Sometimes it was so bad, I just left the trolley and dashed home. I hadn't a clue what to do, so I just made excuses and got other people to do the shopping. It was easy with the baby being so young. I kept it a secret in case people thought I was going mad, but one day I got so desperate I phoned a helpline I got from a magazine. They were so understanding and knew exactly what I was talking about. I couldn't believe it. They even explained to me how to get it sorted out. It was all done over the phone. An absolute lifeline.

Lynn, 30

13

How far you
have come

In this last chapter of Part 3, we show you where you can look forward to being, at the end of your journey through postnatal depression (PND). After you have come through the diagnosis, the treatment and the sometimes painful struggle towards recovery, we assure you that this pot of gold will be there, waiting for you. Never be tempted to give in or give up and let PND win its battle with you. You will win, and you will succeed, so never, ever think about giving up.

Where you will be

Recovering from PND can be a long journey with many twists and turns along the way. For some lucky women, it can be a fairly straight and short road and we really hope that you will be one of those women. It can also take a tremendous effort to hang on in there and keep moving forward despite the bad days and the setbacks. Whatever the road is like for you, you will come to the end of it. Be assured that you will be your old self again, but you will be a wiser self and you'll be a stronger self.

This experience cannot fail to have changed you, but it will have changed you for the better. Struggling through adversity is an unfortunate part of life, which happens to us all at some stage in our lives, and by dealing with these struggles, we can learn so much more about life, and much more about ourselves. We can also understand the difficulties other people are going through all the better and we can recognize these sooner. So we can be there for our friends and loved ones when they need us. They won't need to ask. When you have experienced emotional pain and loss of spirit, you will always know it when you see it in other people, and you will truly be able to empathize, and be there for those people. And that can give you great satisfaction for the rest of your life.

As you recover, you will be surprised by how easily you will slip back into your old routine, or settle into your new one with your baby. You will find that the terrible experience you've had will move slowly and unnoticed out of the forefront of your mind to somewhere much more out of reach. You will never forget it, but you won't think of it every day. Life will resume its old familiarity and be so very comforting for that. Doing ordinary everyday things can feel so joyous and fulfilling when you have just recovered from depression.

If you are on your own

If you have had to come through PND on your own, without a partner, or without close family, you can be especially proud of what you have achieved. Many women have to do this alone, without anyone to support them, and this takes incredible amounts of strength and staying power. You should allow yourself a great sense of achievement for having taken this journey alone, and reached the end of it. Life will be good again for you too. We hope that you have found new friends along the way, who will be around you, giving you support and strength for many days to come. This kind of support is so important.

You and your baby

By this stage, whether you are on your own, or with your partner, you and the new addition to the family should be getting along much better with each other. It may be difficult to remember the bad old days when it was all such a problem and such a source of anxiety, guilt, shame and goodness knows what other feelings. All the pills, or sessions with the therapist, all the bad days, the self-doubt and the low, despairing moods will all be worth it for the feelings of joy and pleasure you will have every day with this wonderful child in your life. If you are still having difficulties with your feelings about the baby, don't be alarmed. You must give it time, and you will get there. There is no set timescale for these things. Keep in touch with some of the organizations you'll find in Part 5 and they will give you useful advice and information to keep you moving in the right direction.

You and your partner

You will have had your ups and downs with your partner, but when PND is in the past, the two of you will be able to be close and secure again. Having come through this huge struggle together will have made you much stronger as a couple. You'll know each other better. You'll have a deeper understanding of each other and what commitment really means. You'll know you can rely on him, no matter what. If your baby was your first with him, you will have adjusted to being a family and not just the two of you and he will have become used to sharing you with the baby. You will have become a family, happy with your life together.

If things have not gone so well, and you are still having difficulties with your relationship, don't be afraid to get some help with mending that, too. PND is a huge pressure for even the strongest relationship to bear without being damaged, but there is so much that you can do to repair this. When you are feeling better, you will have the energy to do something to turn this around. You could make a start by contacting some of the support organizations whose details you'll find in Part 5. There is no need to feel embarrassed about this. PND is an enormous strain on a relationship, and it will affect each couple differently. Many couples will be feeling just as you are, and there are people out there who will completely understand and will be able to show you the way forward.

You and your other children

If you already have children, or step-children, they will be really pleased to see that you are your old self again. They will be so relieved. Amid their hectic young lives, you will have a very important and central place, even though it doesn't seem like that sometimes. All of what has happened in the past few months will have felt very threatening and unsettling to them and they will be much more relaxed now, and this will probably show in their behaviour and general mood. Their schoolwork will probably be picking up too, and you'll see the grades beginning to climb back to where they were.

If things are still not as you would like them with your other children, don't give up, but keep working at it in the ways we've suggested earlier in the book. You can also look for more help and guidance through the support groups or specialist projects and professionals now available in most areas. They will be ready and willing to help you in whatever way they can. Chapter 16, and your local phone book, will give you a starting point for accessing this invaluable support.

Reassurance and motivation for the bad days

You know now that it won't all be plain sailing on your way to recovery and that this is nothing to worry about. It's an unfortunate part of getting better and just another cruel part of having PND. However, every bad day you get through is one less on the road to being yourself again – and this one may be the last one.

Remember to:

- Try to catch a bad day or a setback before it gets hold of you.

- Always be alert to the signs or the circumstances that are likely to lower your mood.

- Avoid too much stress or getting too tired as these can make a setback or bad day much more likely.

- Be on the look out if you've been physically unwell or in the week before a period. These are times when you are more vulnerable.

- Try to always get up and get moving in the mornings, as you can be at a bit of a low ebb then. Getting moving helps dispel that low feeling.

In other words, look after yourself well. You are an important person, and you should take good care of yourself. You have a baby, and maybe other children, who need you to be well for them. You also need to stay well for yourself too.

We've already given you lots of other ideas on coping with the down days and the occasional setbacks in Chapters 3, 8 and 10 – ideas such as thinking positive thoughts, doing something physically active, playing cheerful music and having some extra me-time as well as always having something available to busy your mind when the down moment strikes, like sudoko, craft work, or a good magazine. You can look back at these any time to refresh your memory.

More hints and tips to pick you up and keep you going on the bad days

- Give a friend a ring and meet for coffee, lunch, a walk or a talk – anything that will get you out and get your mind onto something different and more positive.

- Do something for someone else. This can really help. Make that call you've been meaning to make to a friend who's having a rough time, check on an elderly or disabled neighbour, fill that charity bag that's just about to be collected.

- Smiling, or better still laughing, can be a great mood lifter, so have your favourite comedy DVD always to hand, or one of those books full of amusing snippets. If there is a comedy routine that always makes you laugh, that's the one to have in the DVD, ready to go.

- If you have older children, get out an active and fun game and play it with them.

- Read the children an exciting story and do all the voices and actions.

- Put on your favourite keep-fit DVD and get moving. The children can join in too.

- Plant something – anything – some seeds, herbs or bulbs in the house, conservatory or window box or in the garden or greenhouse if you have one. Planting something and watching it grow can really raise your spirits.

- Call or visit a friend or relative who is always upbeat and positive. It definitely rubs off.

Getting your confidence back

There is so much that is positive and wonderful about having a baby. Bringing a little person into the world, being a mother, and all the marvellous warm feelings that can bring. However, having a baby can also make you feel as if you've disappeared. You are now somebody's mother and somebody's partner or wife. Everyone makes a beeline for the baby when they come to see you, or meet you in the street. So even without PND you can lose your confidence and sense of identity. Having PND can make all of that feel ten times worse.

Here are some suggestions to boost your confidence and re-awaken the old you:

- Write a list of all the things you're good at. This doesn't need to be huge things. Read your list every week, and add to it when you can.

- Grow to like yourself – there will never be anyone else quite like *you*.

- No one in the world is as important to your baby as *you*.

- Do something new and different that really appeals to you. The sense of achievement will energize and enthuse you.

- Remember that many people, despite how they appear, are often as unsure of themselves as you are.

- Take it all gradually, one step at a time.

- Walk the walk and talk the talk – even if you're terrified inside. You'll be amazed at how just acting confident can make you feel more confident too. So head up, shoulders relaxed, make eye contact and smile.

- Have a bit of a mini makeover – clothes, make-up, nails or hair. Have a girlie night with some friends and do each other's nails and hair if funds are low. Treat yourself if you can afford it. You deserve it. This will give you a great confidence boost.

I gave birth to three healthy sons over a period of 16 years. They are all grown up now, and I have one gorgeous grandson. I had PND with all three births and I can still remember the numbing tiredness and the complete isolation I felt. I remember one day catching sight of myself in the mirror and realizing that I hadn't been washing my hair and it was a complete mess. I hadn't even noticed. I gradually recovered each time, but I have two suggestions which might help new mothers today. First, enlist the help of a trusted parent, friend or relative before the baby is born, to be around to listen and give you support for the first few months after the birth. And second, after the birth when those around you ask how they can help, you should answer completely honestly and say exactly what you would like them to do for you.

Pat, 54

I had two pregnancies, and births, in three years. It was all very tiring and very busy, but always upbeat. I was never down or anxious. Everyone said I thrived on motherhood. My husband and I then felt our family was complete and he had a vasectomy. Then, six months later, I was stunned to find I was pregnant again. It was such a shock, neither of us could believe it, but it seems that this can happen. At first I was upset, but then I came round to thinking it was meant to be and I became quite enthusiastic. I'm not sure if it was my age or because of it being unplanned, but for the first time I had PND after the baby was born. I had no idea what had hit me. I'd never in my life felt so completely lost and totally out of my depth. Before this happened, I'd always thought that mothers with PND were just not very good mothers. Not any more. My doctor was such a support and let me sound off whenever I saw her as well as arranging treatment for me really quickly. Now, fully recovered, I can't imagine life without my three wonderful children.

Alisha, 41

Getting back to normal

You may feel that getting back to normal is so far away, that you can't even imagine it now, but it will happen one day. You will wake up one morning and feel good about the day ahead. You'll have that contented and relaxed feeling in your tummy, instead of anxiety and butterflies. You'll regain your old energy. You probably won't know when the exact moment was that you felt your old self again, but you'll realize that it's been a week or two since you had any sign of that old enemy, your PND. The world will be a bright cheerful place again. Colours will be more vivid, the sound of laughter will make you smile again, and the feeling of sunshine on your face will make you shiver with pleasure. But best of all, the touch and smile of your baby will give you an indescribable glow inside.

Introducing Parts 4 and 5

It's now time to finish off this part of the book, and move on to Parts 4 and 5. In the first three parts of the book, we explained all about PND, what it is, why you get it, what to do about it, and so on. The final two parts of the book will be a bit different. In Part 4, you will be hearing mainly from other women who have PND. You'll be hearing fuller stories of their experiences and reading their advice and messages of hope, especially written just for you, including messages from one or two celebrities. Part 5 contains contact details for organizations, helplines and websites that you will find helpful, as well as details of other books that you might want to read.

Part 4:
Messages of
Hope and Support

14

Stories and messages
of hope

We are involved in managing Scotland's anti-stigma campaign 'See me' and have a number of trained media volunteers who have first-hand experience of mental health problems including PND. Our messages of hope would be:
'This is much more common than you might think – you are not alone.'
'Recovery happens – healing is possible.'
'Find someone you can talk to. There are lots of self-help groups where people are going through or have suffered similar pain.'
'You don't need to lose yourself in being a mother.'

The Scottish Association for Mental Health (SAMH)

After the birth of my third baby I suffered a severe bout of postnatal depression. During the time I was ill I was in contact with a woman who had had the illness and was better. She could describe symptoms which were like those I was experiencing and yet she was well again. Talking to her was the only thing that made me think I might ever recover.

As I started to get over my illness I realized that there must be thousands of mums like me who had postnatal depression but who suffered in isolation, behind closed doors, often telling only their partner or their doctor, often with little hope of a recovery. To try to remedy this situation, and with the help of three doctors, my supporter and my sister, we founded the Association for Post-Natal Illness. This organization works to help the 70,000 women in the UK who suffer each year from this most distressing illness after giving birth. We have a nationwide network of over 500 volunteers, who have suffered from postnatal depression and are now better, who support women that are currently ill over the phone, by email or by post.

Our staff can offer sufferers and their families information and advice. We make no charges for our services or our publications. I feel very lucky that I have recovered from postnatal depression. I also feel privileged to be involved with the Association and the wonderful people who provide so much help and support to sufferers all over the country, and the generous donors who support the work we do. I would say to anyone who is currently ill, 'Don't despair. You will get better.' I have spoken to thousands of women in the depths of this illness and they are all better now leading happy, busy lives. Postnatal depression is a terrible illness, it strips you of your self-confidence and self-esteem. It affects your emotions so that you feel like a wreck of your former self. Most sufferers feel despair and think that they can never be well again but there is a future and it is bright. I would say to all sufferers, 'You will get better' and I would repeat this again and again.

Clare Delpech

I had a mild PND after the birth of my first child but this was not ever diagnosed (even though I was a mental health nurse at the time!). However, when I had my next baby I was very unwell indeed. I pretty much withdrew from the world, spending days at home with the curtains closed, often staying in bed, even keeping my head under the pillow to avoid the world. This continued for several years at various levels. I think the thing that helped was my own belief that this would pass eventually. It was hell and there were times when I felt my belief wavering and that was when my friends and family had the biggest role to play; in particular my husband. I hung onto his certainty that it would be okay, that he still loved me, that he wasn't giving up on me, and this gave me the freedom to let go of the anxiety of what the future held and just to focus on the day in hand.

I was taking antidepressants which did help but I didn't seem to be able to 'get over the hump' so I eventually went along to my doctor and disclosed some unresolved issues from my difficult childhood. In due course I got support from a psychologist and this was invaluable to me. I slowly began to feel better, more in control than I had for some time as I was confronting and dealing with the underlying issues. I always describe it as being like trying to get a physical wound to heal while there is an underlying infection – it's just not going to happen, you need to sort out the underlying problems (if there are any) to get better. As I worked through my experiences and, more importantly, my feelings and emotions relating to them, I began to slowly improve. Like constructing a building I was setting down more secure foundations for my life. This has meant I have gone from strength to strength. I no longer need medication but still use the strategies I learned from the psychologist and, of course, my fantastic husband is still my number one supporter.

I recently had a serious physical illness and coping with this caused me to feel very vulnerable to depression but fortunately I did not have a relapse. I think this is mainly due to the fact that with physical health you can make the very personal decision about how you choose to react or respond to your situation according to your own personality, but with mental ill health these choices are very compromised as the illness can shatter your perception of who you are and affects your ability to choose your response. Also my recovery is a legacy of the work I did with the psychologist who helped me to build better foundations to cope with the storms of life.

Audrey

I suffered severe PND after the birth of my first child. That was 40 years ago and thankfully there is much more information out there now. It is important to ask for help ASAP. And it will pass. One positive point is that although I suffered PND once, I went on to have two more children and was extremely well after their births. Likewise, my daughter, (herself a doctor) suffered PND after the birth of her second child and was apprehensive about having any more. However, she too had another two children with no problems.

Agnes

To say I suffered from PND may be a bit unfair, but when my son was six months old (I also had a three-year-old daughter) my wife's moods became worse to the extent that one day, during one of the now too often rows, my wife told me she hated the children and left the family home. Over the next few months my wife would only keep in touch by telephone but then gradually she would visit for a few hours.

It took over six months for us to be together again as a family, but we persevered and I am happy to say that we are getting on as well as we ever did. All through this time I kept telling myself that this was not my wife saying these things – it was as if it was a totally different person. And after all, if you love someone, you don't ever give up on them!

Andy

Set yourself small goals or tasks to achieve each day or week and don't be too hard on yourself if you don't achieve every one of them – just concentrate on the ones you did achieve. Even if you don't feel like it, join a mother and toddler group. It may be uncomfortable at first but you'll soon meet other mums who may have experienced similar difficulties. They may be able to give you advice on ways of coping. Even chatting to someone may help you feel less alone.

When I first suffered with Puerperal Psychosis I was in a locked psychiatric ward and felt completely unable to cope with my baby daughter. I was in hospital for six months and at times I thought that my daughter may be taken into care. It was a struggle when I got home but each and every day it got a tiny bit easier and as time passed I developed a fantastic bond with my daughter which I have to this day. She's 13 now and the most precious part of my life.

Eleanor

*My children are now 24, 22 and 19 but I
suffered from what I now know to be
PND with each of them. After each
pregnancy the PND was worse than the
previous time, and eventually it was so
bad that I did try to kill myself as I felt I
just could not cope with the
responsibility of the children. It was
only after this episode that my 'baby
blues' were acknowledged to even exist,
but the help that was available was
pretty minimal by today's standards. I
was told to pull myself together and also
that as a 'daughter of Eve' I
should expect to bring forth my children
in sorrow. Hardly practical advice. I
was also threatened that the children
would be taken from me and put into
care and then put up for adoption if I
did not prove myself as a 'fit mother'.*

*Neither the medical staff nor the
social worker assigned to my case had a
clue what to do and none of them
appeared to be in the least bit interested.
At my GPs (a large general practice
where one never saw the same doctor
twice) there was never any suggestion of*

a referral elsewhere, except that I was admitted to hospital for female sterilization – probably without my informed consent as I didn't sign forms and they were signed for me by a nurse.

Maybe the sterilization was just as well, as I would not have been able to cope with another pregnancy/baby at that time. I had already had three unplanned children due to contraceptive failure (I later found out that because I have coeliac disease the available hormonal contraceptives did not work – although at the time I was found to be at fault for not using them correctly). My husband was as supportive as he could be, but in his late twenties/early thirties he was building his career and his company were less than understanding. He was often away from home for weeks at a time.

When my middle child was born I was discharged from hospital just six hours after the birth (even having had general anaesthetic for complications during the birth) in order to be home for my eldest child, as my husband's company demanded for him to be sent to a factory in Switzerland at less than three hours' notice. I had no family close at hand who could help out. So what did I do? I knew that I needed help and that the help was unlikely to come from any 'official' source, so I placed an advert in a newsagents asking if there were any other new mothers around who would like contact with others in the same situation. After a slow start a group of us started to meet regularly and, as friendships formed, so did babysitting circles and 'collecting from school' services.

I am still in contact with some of the ladies from the group after all this time and after several moves – some internationally. We organized pressure groups to publicize our problems, talking with politicians from all sides of the fence and involving the local press. I'm not sure if we made a lot of difference except that the publicity for our group did result in an increase in our membership and we did get a funding boost.

I still have bouts of depression from time to time but as the years have passed depression has been taken much more seriously and the treatments available have improved beyond all recognition. It certainly isn't perfect but ... would a medic today tell a new mother with PND that she should expect to feel the way she does as 'a daughter of Eve'? I sincerely hope not.

Maria

Postnatal depression can be very frightening; but you do recover. It's important to ask for help from your midwife or health visitor. It is also important to recognize your achievements during your recovery.

Patricia

I think more awareness really is needed. People tend to think if you look okay on the outside then you are okay on the inside. But it's so hard to say anything when everyone is telling you how happy you must be. Don't feel alone, you are not the only one. Keep going.

Jaz

This is for everyone, whether you are suffering from PND or are a partner or family member of someone who has PND. There is definitely light at the end of the tunnel. I was diagnosed with PND four weeks after giving birth to my son in November 2005. My doctor and health visitor only confirmed what I already knew I had. I was totally distraught that after having had such a great pregnancy I had turned into a complete wreck. What had happened to me? I felt a failure, a burden to my husband and my family. I remember constantly thinking I would never get better and would never see Christmas 2005. Thankfully I was prescribed antidepressants and when they eventually worked, which remember takes time, my bad days slowly disappeared. I believe that my recovery was down to a caring family who listened to me day after day encouraging me to stay focused and saying that I would come through it. Also writing down how I felt helped me to focus and see when things were improving. I am due to start back at work next month and the baby is now at nursery – a happy wee bundle of joy. I can honestly say I have more or less returned to my old self. Remember to keep going.

Pauline

Hopefully the message will get out and the stigma will be removed. I'd like to extend a virtual hug to all those suffering with PND and to say you are all doing so well. Although I only get occasional blue days, they are really dark dark blue!

Emily

I cannot explain what it is like to come out of that unexpectedly dark place [PND] which robs you of joy, and into the warmth of understanding. Go on tell someone!

Lucy

The support and counselling that I received when I was finally brave enough to tell someone about how I was feeling have been a massively positive force in our lives. My daughter has had so much fun in the crèche whilst I have been able to let my emotions go in a safe space. This has been invaluable and the help has allowed me to go from depressed mum to happy and positive mum in just six months or so. The thing which scares me most now is recognizing that if it wasn't for this group I probably wouldn't be here today, and that other women are not able to get this type of help. Let's fight to make sure more services become available.

Ann

Our message would be one of hope:
Never give up. Find someone who you
can trust to talk to, and take all the help
you can get. Please don't give yourself a
hard time by feeling guilty and isolated.
You are not the worst mum in the world,
and not the only person feeling the way
you do, even if it seems like it! Admitting
how you feel, the first step, is the hardest
but the most important. After that it
may not be plain sailing the whole time
but you are on the way to getting better.
Go on, break the chains of silence.

CrossReach (Church of Scotland)
Postnatal Depression services in Edinburgh

(Their 'Bluebell Day' campaign raises awareness
of some of the issues around postnatal depression
with a view to helping de-stigmatize the
condition and persuade people to go for help
more quickly.)

I was so unhappy, I used to get a bottle of wine, put credit on my phone and sit at the end of the settee and listen to sad music. I couldn't bear my kids to come near me and used to shout at them and send them away. The house was like a cesspit and everything had got on top of me. It was dirty from moving in and I just couldn't get through and clean it. Everything changed when I met Home-Start: I know I have achieved so much. My volunteer has been so good for me and I know if there's anything I need help with she'll be there for me. We get lots done together and are laughing all the time. She's helped me get into a routine, and I'm keeping on top of things.

I can talk to her about how things were when I was a child, and I'm starting to come to terms with lots of unhappy things. She's very good at listening, she's got a very caring nature. The big turning point was when Home-Start got the local Samaritans Trust to give me a grant to buy carpets and lino. I am so grateful; carpets make your

*room and make you happy. It's not dirty
and dingy any more. I have cleaned and
decorated right through and the curtains
are open; I used to keep them closed
before with everything dark. I've even
felt able to ask the landlord to help with
fencing, repairs etc. I feel I can do this
now because I'm keeping his house nice.
I feel so much better, even though I do
still get some down days. I'm even
thinking about going out to work or
doing some training. I've found myself
and now I like myself. I know I've
achieved so much, all because of
meeting Home-Start.*

Kelly

(Kelly had bad postnatal illness and was not
coping well with her three young children. To
add to her problems her partner had recently left.
She heard about **Home-Start** through an
Education Welfare Officer, and a volunteer from
the charity started visiting her, in her own home.)

I couldn't believe it was happening. We'd planned so carefully, got everything, even created a nursery. No baby was ever more wanted and I sailed through the pregnancy. My sister used to laugh and call me super-mum. I felt euphoric in the labour ward and my husband's face when he saw the baby was something I'll never forget. And then wham! I felt I had fallen into a black hole and there was no way out. I felt too ashamed to tell everyone and I felt a fool after all the boasting that motherhood would be a doddle. Thankfully my mother got the truth out of me and the doctor understood straight away. The health visitor was good too. It took a few months and I knew I was getting better but all the time I worried about the fact that we hadn't really had time to bond. Could I ever make up for that I wondered. Now I sometimes think we're too bonded, she has me around her little finger. I'm now thinking about a brother or sister for her. I know the PND might come back but this time I'll be prepared and I'll know from the start that it can be beaten.

Sarah

Kath's Poem

I want the darkness to consume me
To block out the unending cries.
They chisel their way through my fragile shell
And gnaw away at my feeling soul.

I want to wake up and find her gone
But my dream is never fulfilled.
The innocent perpetrator of the nightmare
remains.
If she won't go, I must.

I falter on the edge of blackness
Countless times I nearly reach my journey's
end.
There will be no void in her life if I am gone.
She thrives without my love.

An uncertain flame quivers in the shadows.
Slowly, too slowly, there is light.
Finally it is bright enough to see again.
And mother and child meet each other at last.

As someone who suffered this condition silently, I felt so alone and at times very frightened of my feelings and emotions. Raising the awareness of just how damaging this condition can be is essential to improve the sanity, and save the lives of both mothers and babies in the UK.

Dawn Breslin
(Confidence coach and author)

In 1989 my son was born. Within a week of his birth I began to experience panic attacks. PND had struck. I lost all interest in my baby and all sense of reality. PND can manifest itself in lots of ways but the worst thing a mother can do to herself is stay silent about the way she feels. There is help out there and you will get better. Talking to other mums who have PND was a great help to me. Despite my success as an actress, I still have days when the darkness clouds over me and I have to stay calm and wait for reality to return. Never lose faith that you will get better. I am delighted to help ensure that mothers no longer have to suffer in silence.

Denise Welch
(Actress and TV presenter)

You are not alone and the sun will shine again and you will feel happy again.

Fern Britton

Part 5:
More Help
at Hand

15

Relaxation and breathing techniques reviewed

In this last part of the book we concentrate on bringing together lots of sources of help for you. We've put them altogether in one place to make them easy to find. In this chapter, we've pulled together all of the relaxation and breathing techniques which have been given earlier, along with advice on how to cope if you have panic attacks. Then, in Chapter 16, you'll find the contact details for numerous organizations, helplines and websites, which you can contact for advice, information and support. There is also a list of other books you might find useful. We finish with some more words of encouragement for you in Chapter 17.

Throughout the book we have suggested many ways of relaxing and breathing to help you to relax and cope better. We have also explained how you can deal with panic attacks. This chapter will bring all of this together again for you, to make it easier to find the instructions when you want to use them or need to refresh your memory.

Take care!

Remember that the techniques given will help you to relax, but they may also reduce your alertness and may even make you feel drowsy. So while working on these and for around ten minutes afterwards, you shouldn't be driving, looking after the baby or operating machinery. You also should be careful not to stand up too quickly.

Relaxation and breathing techniques

1. Scanning
Breathe in while silently scanning your body for any tension.
As you breathe out, relax any tension you found.
Repeat several times.

2. Countdown 1
Focus on your breathing.
Count silently backwards from 10 to 0, saying the next number silently each time you breathe out.

3. Countdown 2
Sit or stand quietly and do a very slow and silent countdown from 10 to 0, and with each downward count, imagine yourself unwinding and letting go a little bit more.
Repeat if necessary.

4. 1-2-3 Breathing
Try this out first when you are already fairly relaxed, until you get a feel for it. Then you can use it regularly throughout each day to keep tension and anxiety at a minimum. You can also use it when you are feeling anxious, to help you to feel better. Sounds simple, but it can be very effective.

Lie or sit with good support.

Let your breath go, then take a gentle breath in to your own slow silent count of 1.........2.........3, then breathe out again in your own time to your own slow and silent count of 1.........2.........3. Continue gently breathing to this rhythm for a minute or two.

5. Total relaxation

Now it's time to try out tensing and relaxing your muscles, to help your body to relax. If you are in any doubt about your physical fitness to try this, check with your doctor. If you still have a wound which is not completely healed, then don't tense that area. If you have raised blood pressure, it is probably better not to try this activity. Stick with the previous methods. Here is what to do.

- Lie or sit comfortably, head supported if possible.

- Deliberately make a fist and tense up both hands really hard for five or six seconds...hold it...now let the tension go.

- Slowly repeat this for each of the following parts of your body in turn:

> – arms
> – shoulders
> – neck and head
> – face
> – back and chest
> – tummy and bottom
> – legs, feet and toes.

- Relax for a few minutes, and enjoy.

- Rouse yourself gradually.

6. Relaxing your mind

The best way to take your mind off your worries is to give it something else to think about, and the way to make your mind relax is to give it something *relaxing* to think about. So let's give this a try. Find a quiet place, where you're not going to be disturbed, try this out and see what works best for you:

- Slow down and relax your body using one of the previous techniques.

- Once relaxed, picture as clearly as you can or focus your mind entirely on any one of these for a few minutes:

- waves lapping on the seashore
- branches swaying in the breeze
- deep dark green velvet
- a word or phrase such as peace, calm, relax
- a calming poem, prayer or picture.

7. Coping with a panic attack

Once you understand the 'fight or flight' reaction, panic attacks can seem much less frightening. However, from a more practical point of view, you need to learn how to deal with them. So, if you have panic attacks, the key is to catch them early and stop them in their tracks. This will put you back in control. Here is one way of doing this, but don't be put off if this method doesn't work the first or even second time you try it. Keep at it. It takes a bit of practice and a bit of determination, but it is very effective. Thousands of people have used it successfully. You can too.

The PAUSE routine

First, work out what your own first signs of a panic attack are. This might be a lurch in the stomach, a thought in your mind, heart rate rising, or something else you've noticed.

Be on the look out for these first signs, and when you notice them, you should immediately:

Pause....and make yourself comfortable (sit down, lean on something etc.)

Absorb....detail of what's going on around you

Use....any method of relaxing quickly which works well for you, *then*

Slowly....when you feel better,

Ease....yourself back into what you were doing.

That's:

P Pause

A Absorb detail around you

U Use relaxation, then

S Slowly,

E Ease yourself back into what you were doing.

16

Useful contacts, websites and books

Useful contacts

Association for Post-Natal Illness (APNI)
145 Dawes Road, Fulham
London SW6 7EB
Tel: 020 7386 0868
email: **info@apni.org**
web: **www.apni.org**

Best time to telephone: 10.00 a.m. to 2.00 p.m., Monday and Friday; 10.00 a.m. to 2.00 p.m. Tuesday to Thursday (answerphone at other times).

Formed in 1979, the APNI offers support for postnatal depression and Postnatal Psychosis. If callers phone when the office is closed and leave a message, APNI will always return their call. Also APNI has a booklet which is free to women who would like more information about postnatal depression.

Aware
72 Lower Leeson Street,
Dublin 2
Tel: (00353) (0)1 661 7211
Helpline (loCall): (00353) (0)1890 303 302
web: **www.aware.ie**

Aware is a voluntary organization formed in 1985, and aims to assist those whose lives are directly affected by depression. Support groups throughout Ireland are available from the website. The helpline is open seven days a week from 10.00 a.m. to 10.00 p.m. From Thursday to Sunday, the helpline also operates after 10.00 p.m.

BLISS

Freephone: 0500 618 140 – family support helpline.
email: **enquiries@bliss.org.uk**
web: **www.bliss.org.uk**

Support for families of premature babies.

The Breastfeeding Network

PO Box 11126,
Paisley PA2 8YB
Helpline: 0870 900 8787
web: **www.breastfeedingnetwork.org.uk**

An independent source of support and information for breastfeeding women and others.

British Association for Counselling and Psychotherapy (BACP)
BACP House,
35–37 Albert Street,
Rugby CV21 2SG
Tel: 0870 443 5252
email: **bacp@bacp.co.uk**
web: **www.bacp.co.uk**

Contact for details of local counsellors and therapists (fee paying).

British Confederation of Psychotherapists (BCP)
West Hill House, Swains Lane,
London N6 6QS
Tel: 020 7267 3626
web: **www.bcp.org.uk**

A network of psychoanalytical psychotherapy societies. It can provide a register of members.

Church of Scotland Post-Natal Depression Project
Wallace House, 3 Boswell Road,
Edinburgh EH5 3RJ
Tel: 0131 538 7288

Best time to telephone: 9.00 a.m. to 5.00 p.m. Monday to Friday.

Locally based project. Individual counselling, therapy groups, some local drop-in centres, telephone support, infant massage.

CrossReach
Charis House,
47 Milton Road East,
Edinburgh EH15 2SR
Tel: 0131 657 2000
email: **info@crossreach.org.uk**
web: **www.crossreach.org.uk**

Cry-sis
BM Cry-sis,
London WC1N 3XX
(please enclose SAE)
email: **info@cry-sis.org.uk**
web: **www.cry-sis.org.uk**

Helpline: 08451 228 669 Available from 9.00 a.m. to 10.00 p.m every day. The answering service will give you the phone number of volunteer contacts, who once had similar problems.

Cry-sis offers support for families with excessively crying, sleepless and demanding babies.

Depression Alliance

Helpline: 0845 120 3746 (weekdays 7.00 p.m. to 10.00 p.m.)

web: **www.depressionalliance.org**

Telephone support for mothers suffering from perinatal (pre- and postnatal) depression, and their families.

Depression Alliance Cymru (Wales),

11 Plas Melin,
Westbourne Road, Whitchurch,
Cardiff CF4 2BT
Tel: 029 2069 2891

Depression Alliance Scotland,

3 Grosvenor Gardens,
Edinburgh EH12 5JU
Tel: 0845 123 23 20
email: **info@dascot.org**
web: **www.dascot.org**

Fellowship of Depressives Anonymous
Box FDAI,
c/o Self-Help Nottingham,
Ormiston House,
32–36 Pelham Street,
Nottingham NG1 2EG
web: **www.depressionanon.co.uk**

Offers information, support and local groups.

Home-Start
Home-Start UK,
2 Salisbury Road,
Leicester LE1 7QR
Freephone: 0800 068 63 68
email: **info@home-start.org.uk**
web: **www.home-start.org.uk**

Informal and friendly support for families with young children. Home-Start's trained volunteers offer friendship and informal support to parents with young children in 345 local communities throughout the UK.

The International Association of Infant Massage
For further information on how to find a baby massage instructor in your area, contact general enquiries on: 07816 289788.

email: **mail@iaim.org.uk**
web: **www.iaim.org.uk**

MAMA

National Meet A Mum Association
54 Lillington Road,
Radstock BA3 3NR
Tel: (helpline): 0845 120 3746 weekdays 7.00 p.m. to 10.00 p.m. (the helpline is run under the auspices of Depression Alliance).
web: **www.mama.co.uk**

Nationwide organization which was launched in 1979. Offers information, one-to-one support and over 70 local support groups.

Manic Depression Fellowship

Castle Works,
21 St George's Road,
London SE1 6ES
Tel: 08456 340 540
web: **www.mdf.org.uk**

Mind

15–19 Broadway,
London E15 4BQ
Tel: 020 8519 2122
Information line: 0845 766 0163, open Monday to
Friday 9.15 a.m. to 5.15 p.m.
email: **contact@mind.org.uk**
web: **www.mind.org.uk**

The English national association for mental
health, which has many local branches.

The National Childbirth Trust (NCT)

Alexandra House,
Oldham Terrace, Acton,
London W3 6NH
web: **www.nct.org.uk**
NCT pregnancy and birth line: 0870 444 8709
NCT breastfeeding line: 0870 444 8708
Enquiry line: 0870 444 8707

NCT is a leading charity for pregnancy, birth and
parenting in the UK. It supports thousands of
people each year, offering relevant information,
reassurance and mutual support. There are over
60,000 members across the UK.

NHS Direct
Tel: 0845 4647
General advice on health matters from the UK's
National Health Service.

No Panic
93 Brands Farm Way,
Randley, Telford,
Shropshire TF3 2JQ
email: **ceo@nopanic.org.uk**
web: **www.nopanic.org.uk**
Free helpline: 0808 808 0545, every day from
10.00 a.m. to 10.00 p.m.

Information and support for panic attacks,
phobias, obsessions.

**Northern Ireland Association for Mental
Health**
Central Office, 80 University Street
Belfast BT7 1HE
Tel: 028 9032 8474 (central office)
web: **www.niamh.co.uk**

OCD Action
22/24 Highbury Grove,
Suite 107,
London N5 2EA

Tel: 0845 390 6232 (help and information line)
email: **info@ocdaction.org.uk**
web: **www.ocdaction.org.uk**

OCD Action is a national UK charity for people with obsessive compulsive disorders.

PMS & PND Support

c/o 113 University Street,
Belfast BT7 1HP
Tel: 028 9065 3209
web: **www.pmspndsupport.co.uk**

PMS & PND Support was founded in 1988 and is a voluntary organization run by sufferers and ex-sufferers of premenstrual syndrome and postnatal depression. It aims to provide support, advice and information to PMS and PND sufferers and their families.

PNi-SHA Perinatal Illness-Support & Help Association

c/o Ashbourne Adult Education Centre
Cockayne Avenue, Ashbourne,
Derbyshire DE6 1JQ
Tel: 01335 347599
email: **help@pnisha.org.uk**
web: **www.pnisha.org.uk**

PNi-SHA is a charitable organization offering information, emotional support and practical help to women and their families affected by any type of antenatal and postnatal illness.

Relate
National Marriage Guidance,
Herbert Gray College,
Little Church Street,
Rugby CV21 3AP
web: **www.relate.org.uk**

Relate offers advice, relationship counselling, sex therapy, workshops, mediation, consultations and support face to face, by phone and through their website.

Samaritans
Tel: 08457 90 90 90 (24-hour helpline)
email: **jo@samaritans.org**

SANE
1st Floor Cityside House,
40 Adler Street,
London E1 1EE
Tel: 0845 767 8000
web: **www.sane.org.uk**

A charity concerned with improving the lives of everyone affected by mental illness. SANE's national telephone helpline offers support and information to callers throughout the UK.

The Scottish Association for Mental Health (SAMH)
Cumbrae House
15 Carlton Court,
Glasgow G5 9JP
Tel: 0141 568 7000
email: **enquire@samh.org.uk**
web: **www.samh.org.uk**

The Scottish association for mental health.

Stillbirth and Neonatal Death Society (SANDS)
28 Portland Place,
London W1N 4DE
Tel: 020 7436 5881 (national helpline)
web: **www.uk-sands.org**

Stresswatch Scotland
Tel: 01563 574144 (helpline) Monday to Friday 10.00 a.m. to 6.00 p.m.)
email: **office@stresswatchscotland.com**
web: **www.stresswatchscotland.com**

Scottish national charity offering advice and support for stress, anxiety, panic and phobias.

United Kingdom Council for Psychotherapy (UKCP)
2nd Floor, Edward House,
2 Wakley Street,
London EC1V 7LT
Tel: 020 7014 9955
Fax: 020 7014 9977
email: **info@psychotherapy.org.uk**
web: **www.psychotherapy.org.uk**

Regional lists of psychotherapists are available free.

Helpful websites

Depression in pregnancy

For women who experience depression during pregnancy.

www.depression-in-pregnancy.org.uk

Discussion/support forum for PND:

www.postnataldepression.org.uk/forums

For fathers

Fathers Direct

The National Information Centre on Fatherhood

News, training information, policy updates, research summaries and guides for supporting fathers and their families.

www.fathersdirect.com

Medication information

Motherisk

A website listing information about drugs in pregnancy and breastfeeding.

www.motherisk.org

NHS

General advice on health matters from the UK National Health Service.

www.nhsdirect.nhs.uk

Parenting

Web-based parenting organization helping parents share information and advice.

www.netmums.com

Postnatal illness website

A self help and mutual support site for sufferers and survivors of postnatal illness and postnatal depression. As well as support for women with PNI/PND the forum offers mutual support for partners, husbands and helpers of women with PNI.

www.pni.org.uk

Relationships

Relate offers advice, relationship counselling, sex therapy, workshops, mediation, consultations and support face to face, by phone and through this website. You can also find your nearest Relate and consult experts online.

www.relate.org.uk

Traumatic childbirth

For women who have experienced traumatic childbirth.

www.birthtraumaassociation.org.uk

Useful books

Antenatal and Postnatal Depression (2000),
  S. Curham (Vermilion).

Coping with Postnatal Depression (2005), Dr Sandra
  L. Wheatley (Sheldon Press).

Fatherhood: The Truth (2005), Markus Berkmann
  (Vermilion).

Life after birth (2000), Kate Figes (Penguin Books).

*Overcoming Depression: A Self-help Guide Using
  Cognitive Behavioural Techniques* (2000),
  P. Gilbert (Constable).

*Parenting Well When You're Depressed: A Complete
  Resource for Maintaining a Healthy Family*,
  (2001) J. Nicholson, A. D. Henry and
  J. C. Clayfield (New Harbinger).

*Relax It's Only a Baby: The No-Fuss Guide to
  Parenting*, (2005) Denise Robertson (Little
  Books).

When Someone You Love Has Depression (2003),
  Barbara Baker (Sheldon Press).

17

Moving on

We have come a long way together from the beginning of the book, when you were feeling so low and searching for answers to so many questions. We do hope that we have answered most of your questions or at least given you the information you need to find the answers if we couldn't provide them here for you. We may not have been able to take your pain away, but at least you know what you are dealing with now, and you know there are people out there who can and will help you.

Your doctor, midwife and health visitor are there for you, and a myriad of people are out there in voluntary groups and charities all over the country, ready to help and support you through this illness. You know that you are not alone any more. Many, many other women are suffering today right now, just the way you are. We are here, too, on your side. You know now that you will get better and you will be your old self again. This very difficult time in your life will pass. We both assure you of that.

What now?

We may be at the end of the book, but this isn't the end of for you. This is only the beginning. This is a new start for you. We hope that from today you will be setting out with renewed energy on your road to recovery. This book will still be here for you in the coming days and weeks. It will be here for you to look back over as you move through different stages, so that you can re-read some sections to refresh your memory as they become more relevant. Our list of support groups, helplines, websites and useful books will always be there to answer any new questions you may have, or when you need to talk to someone. You can dip back into this book when you need its hints and tips for relaxing, coping with panic attacks, staying motivated, coping with the downs, the low moments, the setbacks, massaging your baby, or coming off your medication – and, of course, when you begin to think about adding to your family.

Helping other mothers with PND

When at last you have come through this incredible journey towards recovery, and have emerged safely out the other side, you may feel you could help other mothers who are just setting out on that journey. Many women who have experienced postnatal depression (PND) feel a need to do this, and to speak up so that other women can recognize this distressing illness much sooner, and get the help they desperately need. Women still only thinking about a pregnancy might be able to take steps to prevent PND happening in the first place. There are many hard-working organizations and groups throughout the country who are trying to do this. Reaching out and helping others can help you to feel better too. If you decide you want to give something back to others, and offer your support to any of these organizations, don't hesitate to get in touch with them. When you feel up to it, you'll find all the details in Chapter 16, so there's nothing to stop you. They will welcome you warmly, and appreciate your input, however small.

Good luck

We know that it may be difficult for you to imagine a brighter future at the moment, but we promise you that it is out there, waiting for you. All you need to do is to begin putting your trust in someone who can help get you through this. Allow yourself to share this burden with someone who understands how heavy it is to carry all by yourself and, when you do, you will be so much stronger for the experience. It has been a privilege to be able to write this book for you, and we wish you and your family all the luck in the world, and all the happiness too. You deserve it.